A Guide to
Patient Recruitment and Retention

Diana L. Anderson, Ph.D.

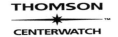

THOMSON
CENTERWATCH

22 Thomson Place · Boston, MA 02210
Phone (617) 856-5900 · Fax (617) 856-5901
www.centerwatch.com

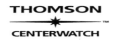

A Guide to Patient Recruitment and Retention
by Diana L. Anderson, Ph.D.

Editor	**Design**
Sara Gambrill	Paul Gualdoni, Jr.

Copyright© 2004 by CenterWatch, a division of Thomson Healthcare, Inc. Thomson Healthcare™ is a trademark used herein under license.

Printed in the United States.
  2 3 4 5 07 06 05

For more information, contact CenterWatch, 22 Thomson Place, Boston, MA 02210. Or you can visit our Internet site at http://www.centerwatch.com.

ISBN 1-930624-45-X

FOREWORD

Developing and gaining expertise in the field of patient recruitment and retention is a constant challenge in an ever changing landscape. I have personally spent 12 years trying to figure out how to fine tune the nuances of this critical aspect of the clinical trials business. I engage with a team that continuously works to streamline and improve processes to address the many variables we encounter as we strive to deliver positive outcomes to our clients.

Overall the clinical trials business is complex, with many players and stakeholders, all of whom are ultimately dependent upon the investigative site to perform. Patient recruitment and retention are no exception. Like any other aspect of the clinical trials arena, delivering positive outcomes is certainly not a game of chance. In addition, as with many of the marketing-related strategies we employ, what we do is not totally based in science, but a balance between art and science. For example, over time we have come to understand that media and communications are only part of the solution contributing to a successful recruitment/retention program. Although media buying and management of media are only part of the more concrete aspects of our business, they prove to be a continuous challenge, considering that we are "selling" a "product" to a population of individuals who for the most part have never heard of a clinical trial!

It appears that the future may bring us back to what I consider "the basics" of patient recruitment and retention. These principles include the blending of site-focused, site support recruitment/retention strategies combined with marketing/communication expertise, which is where the art and science of our work come together. Building a relationship of understanding with our customers—the investigative site and the consumer/participant in the clinical trial process—is the ultimate goal.

I have heard discussions over the years that what we "do" in this niche is not rocket science; I beg to differ. Providing a service to the pharmaceutical industry such as patient recruitment and fulfilling a commitment to deliver satisfaction are two of the loftiest goals I have ever strived to achieve. We are far beyond the old adage, "50% of marketing works; the challenge is that we don't know which 50%," but we still have much to learn.

The contributors to this book have also, in many instances, dedicated their careers to understanding and developing an area that is beyond infancy, but still in a growth stage. I strongly believe that this new book will be helpful in expanding our knowledge base and strengthening our profession.

ACKNOWLEDGMENTS

I would like to acknowledge a number of contributors to this second book focusing on the field of patient recruitment. First, and most importantly, I would like to thank my colleagues and friends who freely shared their knowledge and experiences. Obviously, without these contributors, the book would not have been possible. The wealth of knowledge about this segment of our industry has grown tremendously since the first book as it has matured. While the concept of patient recruitment was in its infancy when the first book was written, it has come of age now with the second.

Sincere thanks to Ken Getz who believed in the concept of another book, not just a second edition, but a new body of knowledge. He has consistently promoted and understood the importance of patient recruitment/retention to the clinical trials industry. Also deep appreciation to Sara Gambrill from CenterWatch, who has been incisive and supportive throughout our editing process over the last year.

Fortunately for me, there is someone who is always behind the scenes quietly burning the midnight oil by my side, and is a true partner in many of my personal successes. Susan Golladay, who works with me in the role of Executive Assistant, has contributed to managing administrative activities, word processing, author communication and many other tasks related to the book. She has also helped keep the book "with me" no matter where I have been over the last year, and that has been a challenge!

I think I can speak for all of us, Ken, Sara and Susan, when I say that we hope those who read and use the book will be as excited as we are with what we have to share, and that the information will help provide value to support your efforts.

Sincerely,
Diana L. Anderson

TABLE OF CONTENTS

Table of Contents

PART ONE

Current Landscape and Planning

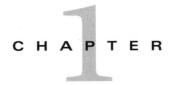

C H A P T E R

The Patient Recruitment Market: A History and Overview of Today's Issues

Diana L. Anderson, Ph.D., D. Anderson & Company

Objectives
- Identify the challenges in accelerating patient recruitment
- Highlight the importance of patient retention
- Delineate scientific aspects of patient recruitment such as market research and outcomes metrics
- Describe new approaches in patient recruitment such as using preferred recruitment providers, and making patient recruitment a core competency for study monitors

Introduction

Patient recruitment efforts are becoming increasingly sophisticated to accommodate enrollment demands linked to the rising number of global clinical trials. Active investigational new drug applications (INDs) are approaching 4,000 per year (Table 1), the number of subjects per NDA currently exceeds 5,300 (Table 2), and approximately 80,000 clinical trials are ongoing in the United States alone.[1] Attracting, enrolling and retaining study subjects in many of these trials is a challenge, and meeting that challenge successfully in accordance with established timelines requires well-designed initiatives by trained staff or professional recruitment providers.

The days of sponsors' simply handing lump sums of recruitment funds to investigative sites and hoping they use it to develop a successful recruitment campaign are numbered. In today's competitive market, "hoping" for

Table 1: Active Clinical Studies

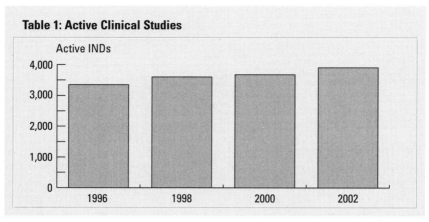

Source: PhRMA, FDA, 2003

Table 2: Average Number of Patients per NDA

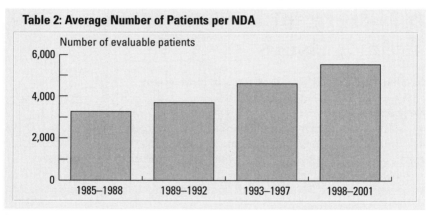

Source: Tufts Center for the Study of Drug Development, 2002; *Food Drug Law Journal*, 1997.

success is not a viable option,[2] especially at a time when more than half of U.S. clinical trials experience enrollment delays of between one and six months.[3] Unstructured attempts at recruitment are being replaced by carefully researched plans that pinpoint which investigators and sites are best suited for a particular study, where the likely study volunteers are, how to reach them, how to remove barriers to study participation, and how to retain candidates. And as studies progress, success of the recruitment efforts is more likely to be measured on a continual basis, allowing for the development of metrics. With the ongoing collection of metrics to measure efficacy, recruitment strategy becomes more scientific and evidence-based. As a result, the likelihood of reaching enrolling targets and the cost per enrolled patient will become more predictable and less of a guessing game.

Keeping metrics is one of several trends gaining a foothold in the realm of professionalized patient recruitment, along with the use of market research, centralized call centers, centralized multi-media campaigns developed by recruitment providers, an improved informed consent process and use of good customer service techniques to enhance patient retention. The goal of taking a professional approach is to accelerate the recruitment process and improve retention in an ethical, fiscally responsible manner.

A Brief History

The clinical development process depends upon successful and ethical patient recruitment practices that are acceptable to the sponsor and the selected institutional review board (IRB). While always critically important to the success of a project, patient recruitment has traditionally received lower priority, particularly when studies were largely conducted at academic medical centers where the thinking was that large numbers of potential subjects were readily available. That thinking has carried over to the present day, as dedicated and part-time sites with their own large databases of patients have entered the picture. Recruitment was and still is often considered the responsibility of the investigative site's study coordinator, typically a healthcare professional with little or no marketing expertise.

With busy study coordinators at the helm, recruitment approaches have often been generic in nature, meaning that similar recruiting techniques were used for most therapeutic areas. For example, recruitment tactics for a diabetes trial might be the same as those used for a migraine headache study. Sponsors glossed over recruitment strategies in favor of protocol adherence, data collection and regulatory issues. They considered the finding of study volunteers to be the site's responsibility. This thinking was reflected in the fact that study budgets negotiated with the site often did not contain a line item for patient recruitment.

In the early 1990s, some of the more experienced investigative sites began to recognize that strategic marketing and advertising campaigns were necessary, and those costs could not be squeezed from the study budget, which had already been allocated to perform other activities of study conduct. Yet, sponsors were reluctant to provide specified recruitment funds at least 50% of the time. The sentiment was, "We've agreed on a study budget, and that should cover the cost of recruitment efforts." By 1993, the sponsors' rate of refusal had dropped to approximately 25%. By 1994, sophisticated sites were developing proposals, including budgets, for sponsors that detailed how recruitment dollars would be used. They had also begun requesting and receiving additional funds, if needed, during the course of the trial.

In the mid-1990s, professional recruitment groups started aggressive marketing of their services, and by 1996, site management organizations (SMOs) were developing full-scale recruitment programs supervised by staff dedicated for this purpose.[4]

Professionalizing Recruitment and Retention

Since the early 1990s, there have been remarkable changes in approaches to patient recruitment and retention. Rudimentary recruiting methods have given way to the development of professional, well-orchestrated strategies led by dedicated staff at larger independent sites, site management organizations (SMOs), some academic medical centers and patient recruitment providers. At the same time, sponsors have begun to understand the need for procedures to support patient recruitment initiatives, and are investing significant resources in the development of staff and programs internally to provide recruitment services. Therefore, the environment now includes those that focus on recruitment within the pharma companies themselves in addition to external outsourcing partners, who provide centralized recruitment partners.

CenterWatch estimates that in 2002, $500 million were spent on mass media promotion, up from $400 million just two years earlier.[5] According to CenterWatch, these figures represent dollars allocated to central campaigns and to individual site initiatives.

With so much at stake, spending dollars wisely, productively and ethically is at the heart of the recruitment industry, which is dedicated to meeting or beating enrollment targets in the allotted time frame. Efforts to meet this goal have resulted in centralized media campaigns orchestrated by domestic and international recruitment vendors, expanded use of centralized call centers, discussion of patient recruitment plans at investigator meetings, market research and more. A single multi-center campaign may use some or all of these modalities to attract the required number of volunteers.

Professional recruitment providers often work with sponsors, contract research organizations (CROs), and site management organizations (SMOs) to enhance recruitment efforts at the site level, where recruitment and enrollment actually occur. These companies can structure entire media packages, including the design and placement of advertising, detailed follow-up, fine-tuning of strategy as the project unfolds and development of metrics to document efficacy.

Recruitment providers are a valuable resource, as many investigative sites lack staff and expertise in recruitment strategy. Recent data suggest that more than one-third of all investigative sites conduct research on a part-time basis (Table 3).[6] Generally, these are the sites that are not positioned to undertake targeted recruitment campaigns when they need to reach beyond their internal patient database to reach enrollment goals—something that happens nearly half the time.[7] Furthermore, it is unlikely that they can justify dedicating a staff member to recruitment tasks, meaning that this vital activity either falls through the cracks or is tacked onto the responsibilities of the study coordinator who is probably already overburdened.

Table 3: Market Share of Industry-Sponsored Clincal Trials by Site Type

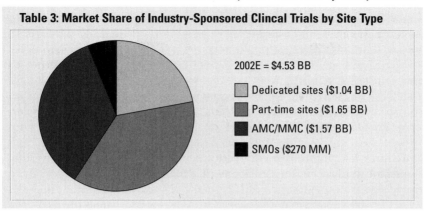

2002E = $4.53 BB

☐ Dedicated sites ($1.04 BB)
⬛ Part-time sites ($1.65 BB)
⬛ AMC/MMC ($1.57 BB)
⬛ SMOs ($270 MM)

Source: Tufts Center for the Study of Drug Development, 2002; *Food Drug Law Journal*, 1997.

Dedicated sites, SMOs and the more organized academic medical centers (AMCs) may have internal recruitment capability, but they can still benefit from professional intervention. Tasks such as developing media campaigns for multiple trials; placing advertising; telephone pre-screening; scheduling of appointments; and mailing out of brochures explaining the clinical trials process, disease-specific flyers, and reminder cards for upcoming appointments are enormously time consuming, and may prove too overwhelming for a one- or two-person operation.

Centralized recruitment efforts can also assist sites in focusing greater attention on patient retention. Too often, efforts focus almost exclusively on recruitment, but retention is just as important because on average, nearly one-quarter of study volunteers drop out before completing the study.[8] Every time a study subject drops out, another one must be recruited, enrolled and randomized, certainly a costly, time-consuming exercise, and one that can be minimized through improved retention efforts.

Retention of study subjects should be viewed as a direct reflection of how much they understand about the clinical trials process and the importance of protocol adherence. Educating study volunteers about the process in which they are about to engage, explaining their responsibilities to them as study candidates and always showing respect for them increases their sense of buy-in and should improve retention.

David Scott, Vice President of Palm Beach Research Center (PBRC), says that ongoing education of the study volunteers is part of PBRC's informed consent process. "We like to think that informed consent is a process that lasts until the patient completes the study. Fully informing the patient along the way as to what will happen at each visit keeps them more in the loop, and hopefully will result in their staying in the study until the end," Scott comments.

Retention of study volunteers is linked to how valued they feel, and how well they are treated at each point of contact, from their first phone screen, to the first screening visit, to regular study visits throughout the trial. These are elements of good customer service and current thinking supports the notion that essentially, study volunteers want to be treated like customers.

As customers, they expect trials to be convenient. One survey revealed that among participants who had considered participating but ultimately opted not to, convenience-related issues weighed heavily. In fact, "center was too far away," and "inconvenient hours" ranked substantially ahead of concerns about receiving placebo (Table 4).

Table 4: Reasons for Not Participating in a Clinical Trial

■ Unable to find a trial	57%
■ Not eligible	39%
■ Center was too far away	37%
■ Inconvenient center hours	26%
■ Not enough information	12%
■ Concern about getting placebo	9%

Source: CenterWatch, 2002

Considering participation in a study is different from staying in a study once enrolled, but the two are connected as part of a continuum of interaction with study subjects. Sites need to be educated as to the importance of this interaction so they become aware of the importance of taking steps as simple as calling pre-screened candidates in a timely fashion to schedule the first visit. Nearly one-quarter of pre-qualified volunteers fail to randomize because they never receive follow-up calls from the site. Another 14% lose interest once they do interact with the site.[9] Anecdotal data suggest that if a pre-qualified candidate is not scheduled within three to five days for a first appointment, there is a high likelihood that the individual will lose interest.[10] There is a wealth of resources able to help offer solutions (Table 5). However, whoever provides support and where, the core of all recruitment solutions ultimately rests with the investigative site participation and follow-up with recruitment efforts.

Table 5: Some Patient Recruitment Providers

Name	Type
Acurian	Customized data mining of proprietary databases of individuals who have opted in
AmericasDoctor	Develops customized programs through ADvantage Patient Recruitment; central call center
BBK Healthcare	Produces tailored recruitment campaign solutions
D. Anderson & Co.	Creates targeted recruitment campaigns using market research; Best Recruitment Practices© training program
Essential Patient Recruitment	Uses PAR (Patient Acquisition and Randomization) Funnel, a proprietary forecasting tool, to meet enrollment goals
GCI Group	Combines healthcare communications with state-of-the-art technology solutions
Healthcare Communications Group	Integrates targeted media with community outreach; certified sites
Integrated Clinical Trial Services	Integrated approach using advertising, media services, education programs, concept design and trial branding
MMG	Customized patient recruitment strategies; central call center
Medici Group	Comprehensive strategy for patient recruitment process
MCCI Patient Recruitment	Recruitment campaigns and graphic development
NTegra	Recruiter that guarantees enrollment
Pharmaceutical Research Plus	Accelerated Patient Recruitment System uses comprehensive approach
PharmaTech Solutions	Patient Management Organization (PMO) that uses analysis of potential patient population
Praxis Communications	Centralized patient recruiting, fulfillment center
Verispan	Product Accelerator uses claims data to improve site identification
Veritas Medicine	Online resource that facilitates prospective patients' access to clinical trial information

A Word About Metrics

Metrics are heading toward center stage as patient recruitment initiatives become more scientific. This is a significant change from the 1990s when the practice of keeping metrics was very much in its infancy. At that time, there were few benchmarks and a limited body of literature dedicated to recruitment. In an industry where formal budgeted recruitment efforts have historically taken a back seat to laissez-faire recruiting practices and in-house database screening, metrics have been either nonexistent or amounted to little more than counting the number of calls generated from various advertisements. Their approach is no longer accepted by sponsors that are paying the bills, nor should it be.

With increasing pressure to accelerate clinical timelines, more dollars are flowing into recruitment. And with them comes the understanding that recruitment success has to be measured, and that accountability is destined to become standard practice. Accountability involves a complete tracking of each point of contact, starting with the pre-screening call through to scheduling of the first screening visit, recruitment, enrollment and retention, then linking these actions to the referral source. Through continuous measurement of these actions, meaningful metrics will take shape.

With a metrics-driven recruitment practice, it will eventually be possible to develop substantial therapeutic-specific data useful in predicting outcomes with relative certainty. Using this approach, the emphasis will and has shifted from calculating the number of enrolled patients needed per month toward a more proactive upfront prediction as to whether the enrollment timeline will be met (Table 6).[11]

Table 6: Clinical Trial Enrollment Forecasting	
Today	**Future**
We need two patients per site per month to meet our enrollment timeline.	Metrics suggest that there is an 80% probability of hitting our enrollment timeline.

Source: DIA session, 2003

While sponsors, sites and recruitment vendors work to refine their metrics tracking and reporting systems, simple tools can facilitate the assessment of recruitment performance effectiveness. The "Leaky Pipe" analysis provides a visual display of where along the recruitment–retention continuum the majority of patients are being lost. This diagnostic tool can quickly help to identify the most appropriate interventions needed to adjust a recruitment program. As illustrated in Figure 1, the majority of candidates are being lost during the pre-screening phase.[12] This may suggest that the awareness message or eligibility criteria outlined in the awareness program are so broad that candidates cannot determine for themselves that they would not be eligible for study participation. Based on this assessment, the recruitment team may consider modifying the message before continuing with any additional advertising programs. Alternatively, the Leaky Pipe analysis may reveal a reasonable or expected patient loss through the pre-screening and screening processes but a larger than expected loss through the informed consent process. This would dictate an alternate intervention geared either towards modifying the informed consent document or providing additional training of staff involved in the informed consent process, for example. In this instance, additional advertising or recruiting efforts may not be appropriate as "filling the pipeline" without "fixing the leaks" may not result in the desired increase in randomized patients. Monitoring the flow of patients through the pipeline and assessing whether the "leaks" lessen in response to specific interventions provide a quick determination of the effectiveness of the various interventions.

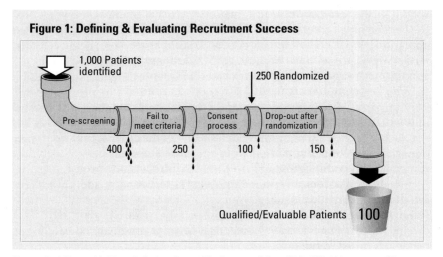

Figure 1: Defining & Evaluating Recruitment Success

Source: Beth Harper, Liz Moench: Patient-Focused Performance Driven Clinical Trial Management™

Eventually, metrics will play a role in retention efforts by predicting and profiling the types of patients most likely to remain in a study, and identifying the techniques and media mix best able to create those results. Predictable success is the promise of metrics—a goal that may not be totally realized for a number of years. Defining and measuring indicators over time are the vehicles for getting there and for ensuring that effective recruitment solutions are designed.[13]

Central Call Centers

Larger investigative sites and SMOs are likely to employ dedicated recruitment staff, but small, part-time or new sites are often left treading water when it comes to recruitment. Trying to fit lengthy telephone screens into a packed work schedule is a challenge that results in calls going unreturned, calls given short shrift, or calls returned at the expense of other pressing tasks. Rather than leaving sites to fend for themselves with volumes of pre-screening calls, sponsors are increasingly turning to central call center services. Recent data point to an upswing in spending on central call centers, with annual growth in the low double digits, reaching an estimated $120 million in 2003.[14]

As the name suggests, a central call center refers to a central switchboard as the destination for all calls for a particular study sourced from advertising and web sites. The caller is screened in a preliminary fashion, and if he or she pre-qualifies for a particular study, the call is forwarded to the appropriate site for further evaluation, or in some cases, a first appointment is scheduled by the screening center. If the call is referred, the site's goal is to schedule an appointment with the potential patient as soon as possible. Some call centers, such as Iris Global Clinical Trial Solutions, can even schedule the appointment at point of patient contact (see Chapter 16).

The key components needed for good centralized recruiting are well-written, highly specific phone screen sheets (Table 7), and the use of trained individuals who can read between the lines to make a determination about the quality of the patient on the telephone. Does the caller sound like someone who is interested in participating in a trial? Does this person seem like someone who is willing and able to comply with the study protocol?

In addition to focusing on inclusion/exclusion criteria, does the screening sheet contain additional rule-out questions, such as concomitant medications, surgeries, recent participation in other clinical trials, etc.? This careful process may raise the percentage of solid pre-qualified candidates being forwarded to the site.

In today's sophisticated market, some call centers have offerings beyond pre-screening. Phone Screen is a central call center offering recruitment, retention and data support services. In 2000, the company launched its Online Reporting capability, which publishes project statistics to a secured web site for instant online viewing by a project sponsor. Online reporting enables sponsors to see up-to-the-minute metrics, such as patient referrals, disqualification reasons, media response and media costs at any time. The information is automatically updated after each phone call, and it can be shared with other team members supplied with appropriate passwords. The company also offers Interactive Voice Response Systems (IVRS), multi-lingual operators, and trend analysis, which tracks the number of days between a patient's pre-qualification by Phone Screen and his or her first appointment at the research site. The sponsor uses these data to identify which sites are handling incoming patients with the greatest efficiency.

Table 7: Segment of a Well-Written Telephone Screen Sheet

IRB Approval Date: _____

Introduction:

Thank you for calling regarding the Type II diabetes research study.

How did you hear about this clinical research trial?

☐ Newspaper

Screener: If newspaper is indicated, please ask for the name of the newspaper.

_____

☐ Radio

Screener: If radio is indicated, please ask name of station.

_____

☐ Brochure

☐ Poster

☐ Other _____

Now, I need to ask you several questions to determine whether you pre-qualify as a potential participant for this Type II Diabetes clinical research trial. All information will be kept strictly confidential and will not be made available to any mailing services.

Name:_____

Address:_____

City:_____State:____Zip:_____

Phone (H): (____)_____-_____ (W): (____)_____-_____

Male/Female:_____ Date of Birth:_____

To qualify for the study, this individual must be between the ages of 18 and 79.

Inclusion/Exclusion Criteria

1. Have you been diagnosed with Type 2 Diabetes? ☐ Yes ☐ No
Screener: If YES, proceed to question 2. IF NO, STOP INTERVIEW.
At this time, you do not qualify for this particular study, since you don't have a diagnosis of Type 2 Diabetes.

2. Are you currently treating your diabetes through diet and exercise? ☐ Yes ☐ No
Screener: IF YES, proceed to question 2a. IF NO, please proceed to Question 3.

2a. Have you had any significant changes in your diet or exercise in the previous 60 days? ☐ Yes ☐ No
Screener: IF YES, STOP INTERVIEW. At this time, you do not qualify for this particular study, since you have had significant changes in your diet and/or exercise. IF NO, proceed to question 3.

3. What medications are you currently taking?_____

Inclusion/Exclusion criteria met at this point: ☐ Yes ☐ No

Patient to be referred to study coordinator: ☐ Yes ☐ No

ClinPhone, based in the United Kingdom, uses interactive voice response (IVR) and interactive web response (IWR) services to enable prospective subjects to pre-screen in 70 languages for studies in some 80 countries. While the company does not have call center capability, it sometimes partners with call centers seeking access to ClinPhone's IVR technology, in an effort to accelerate the screening process. David Stein, Director of Strategic Business Development, explains, "If a call center is fielding calls from several thousand prospective candidates, each taking fifteen minutes, it might be more cost effective for that call center to get the candidate's name and telephone number and ask just a few key questions. If the candidate passes those preliminary questions, he or she would be forwarded to our IVR system for the screen. This approach takes a lot of the burden off of the call center, and saves the sponsor money."

ClinPhone sends e-mails and/or faxes to the investigative sites, advising them that candidates have passed the IVR screen, and the site is to log on to the system or call a toll-free number to get details for follow-up. The company can track in real time which sites are prompt in retrieving data from the system, and can forward those data to the sponsor.

As a trial progresses, ClinPhone offers real-time web, e-mail and fax reports to enable sponsors to measure the success of advertising campaigns, and the number of screen passes against set metrics. If too many or too few prospects are passing the screener, it can quickly be modified using IVR technology which allows for the rapid switching on or off of question modules.

Market Research

In the traditional patient recruitment model, sponsors relied on investigators with proven track records for recruiting an agreed upon number of patients from their own resources. In years past, this approach was generally successful as there were far fewer trials than there are today. With the number of studies growing steadily, sought-after investigators often exhaust their databases as sources of potentially qualified study volunteers and turn to recruitment campaigns.

Sponsors are just beginning to recognize this reality, which challenges their long-held expectation that investigators will be able to achieve all or most of the enrollment target from in-house databases, requiring little or no additional marketing effort. This raises the question as to what sort of efforts are most effective in spurring timely patient enrollment. Broad-based multimedia patient recruitment campaigns can be developed, but before allocating big dollars, sponsors are increasingly using market research to understand which techniques attract the types of patients needed for specific studies.

Market research is a way of finding out what people believe, think, want, need or do. Original or "primary" market research employs systematic, objective techniques to obtain this information, which may not be available through existing or secondary resources. The collected data are analyzed and then used to support decision making and judgment by providing a basis in fact (Table 8). The purpose of conducting market research is to reduce risk in product or service development, thereby increasing likelihood of success.[15]

Table 8: The Market Research Process

- Defining marketing problems and opportunities
- Set objectives, budget and timetables
- Select research types, methods and techniques
- Design research instruments
- Collect the data
- Organize and analyze the data
- Present and use market research findings

Source: www.onlinesbc.gov

Patient recruitment initiatives rooted in market research are inching toward greater acceptance because its scientific basis resonates with sponsors and investigators. Bill Gwinn, Director of Clinical Trial Solutions at Medstat, a healthcare information company, says market research is becoming an integral part of patient recruitment. "There is a profound paradigm shift happening with the industry. Sponsors are starting to use market research, particularly market segmentation—a statistical approach that has long been recognized in the consumer goods industry—as a key to reaching targeted consumer groups."

Market segmentation is the process of dividing a large market into subsets of customers with common characteristics or common needs (Table 9). Segments are developed in two ways: *a priori*—that is, without benefit of primary market research, and involve natural segmentation such as women vs. men, young vs. old, rich vs. poor; or *post hoc*—that is, following multivariate analysis of primary research. Once subsets are defined, marketing efforts can be developed to appeal to market segments of interest, each responding differently to promotions, communications, and advertising.[16]

Table 9: Variables That Segment a Market

- *Demographic*—age, gender, ethnicity, education level, etc.
- *Geographic*—city, state, zip code, census tract, urban or rural, etc.
- *Psychographic*—attitudes, lifestyle, hobbies, risk aversion, etc.
- *Behavioral*—brand loyalty, usage levels, benefits sought, etc.

Source: www.dssresearch.com

Gwinn comments, "In applying market segmentation techniques to patient recruitment initiatives, sponsors gain access to statistics about the media behavior of clusters of patients they are interested in recruiting. Sponsors or recruitment providers on their behalf then use those statistics to develop targeted media campaigns." At Medstat, the clusters are defined through the use of PRIZM, a neighborhood target marketing system that creates the clusters based on a variety of socioeconomic and lifestyle variables.

Multimedia campaigns to the targeted clusters follow primary research that pinpoints candidates in geographies with high prevalence of the diseases of interest. In addition, high prevalence areas are matched to investigators reporting a high volume of office visits from patients with those illnesses.

These sorts of data-driven analyses are quantitative and can have predictive value. There is also qualitative market research, which provides more of an understanding of attitude, perception and opinion. Focus groups and one-on-one interviews are often used in qualitative research because they are, by nature, a structured open discussion providing an exchange of ideas and opinions. Discussion tends to be free flowing, and may be spurred by open-ended questions.

In the drug industry, a sponsor might want to use focus groups with a targeted population to uncover opinions of specific advertisement messages being designed for an upcoming recruitment campaign. Reactions to Advertisements A, B, C and D could be tallied. Generally, this type of qualitative research is not considered to be statistically projectable to the larger targeted population, but is useful to understand attitude.

Whether market analysis is quantitative or qualitative, it is this kind of sophisticated approach that sponsors are seeking to bring substantial improvements to recruitment challenges.

Some Newer Ideas and Regulatory Developments

As call centers and market research gain credibility as tools with positive impact on patient recruitment, other fresh ideas are springing up in the marketplace. These ideas include steps taken by pharmaceutical sponsors to increase their direct involvement in patient recruitment, introducing more scientific principles into patient recruitment and retention, making effective recruitment a core competency for clinical research associates and pushing recruitment to the point of care.

In terms of efforts to improve recruitment outcomes by pushing recruitment to the point of care, John Needham (see Chapter 10) believes that patient recruitment is most effective when the potential subject's physician suggests a study or is the investigator for a study that might benefit that subject. "If a migraine patient is not getting better, and that patient's physician tells her about a potentially helpful migraine study, she might be more inclined to consider screening for it, whether or not her physician is the investigator. So, it's not always about adding more sites or other external strategies, it's about a physician talking to a patient," explains Needham.

There are data to support the notion that potential study volunteers want their physicians involved in their decisions to participate in a clinical trial. In 2002, an online survey of nearly 1,000 participants showed that 73% of respondents want their physicians involved in the decision-making process.[17] Furthermore, once enrollment occurs, about half of those patients prefer to be treated by their own physicians during the trial, highlighting the importance of the doctor–patient relationship as a recruitment and retention technique (Table 10).

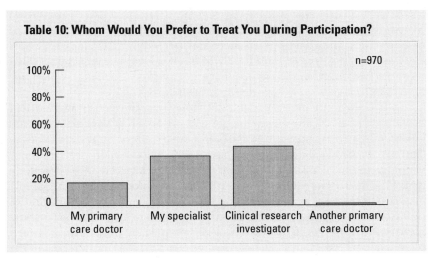

Table 10: Whom Would You Prefer to Treat You During Participation?

n=970

Source: CenterWatch Survey, 2002

Another new trend emphasizes formal training of clinical professionals in patient recruitment techniques. Too often, site staff with recruitment responsibilities learn to develop campaigns in an on-the-job, haphazard way, without the benefit of training or understanding of the importance of upfront planning and metrics. Waiting until recruitment is in rescue mode is too late to begin formulating a plan. These are steps that should be taken at the very beginning of the clinical development process.

D. Anderson & Co., a recruitment provider, has launched the Best Recruitment Practices© training program, a two-day session for recruitment staff, project managers, site directors and CRAs, to develop competencies in recruitment and retention. The program focuses on resource planning, creative media design, working with third-party vendors and site feasibility (assessing site resources to determine enrollment projections realistically). Armed with this information, sites can begin to structure more targeted campaigns.

Jim Kremidas, of Eli Lilly and Co.'s Clinical Trial Enrollment Services, says that major sponsors are expanding recruitment capability in-house. At Eli Lilly, Kremidas heads a central group that provides support to study teams in identifying appropriate interventions for each trial, based on the protocol design, the countries in which the study will take place, and the available budget. "The central group is capturing knowledge continuously about the impact of study design and communication tools across a wide variety of trials and therapeutic areas to help us do our job more effectively. This will include better selection of providers and types of media for specific trials. The knowledge will be contained in a database that Lilly intends to build to help predict effectiveness of different types of recruitment tools," Kremidas explains. "We think that collecting data around the performance of the many tools that one could use to accelerate enrollment is key to making decisions about which tools are most appropriate for a given study."

As part of that effort, Kremidas says his group has already developed metrics showing that in individual studies, various supplier interventions based on those data have proven successful. According to Kremidas, there is a greater appreciation within Eli Lilly of the need for data to support decision making around enrollment, and a raised awareness that there are multiple ways to accelerate enrollment to hit timelines.

One of the more innovative trends involves making patient recruitment proficiency a core competency of the clinical research associate's (CRA's) job. Merck & Co. launched this type of initiative in 2001. According to Susan Tempest, Pharm.D., Site Implementation and Training Manager, this innovation grew out of a recognition that the monitor's job entailed more than reviewing data. "The monitor's role at Merck began changing from that of a data manager to a site manager. This required a review of job competencies needed to perform the new role effectively, and coincided with our interest in supporting our research sites with their recruitment efforts. So, we opted to enhance the skill set of the field monitors in this area, as they are on the front lines." As part of this pilot-stage initiative, Merck's monitors, known as medical research associates, or MRAs, receive recruitment training starting with the concept that the company and the site are forming an alliance to facilitate a successful trial.

MRAs ensure that a recruitment plan is in place, and once the study begins, adherence to present objectives is monitored regularly. Tempest says the idea is to be proactive in terms of recruitment, and not wait until two weeks before the end of the enrollment period to recognize that current strategies will not lead to a site enrolling the targeted number of subjects within the designated enrollment period. Investigative sites that are more sophisticated in terms of their recruitment abilities may require less intervention than sites that are struggling.

Regardless of the amount of recruitment support needed by specific sites, this type of approach encourages more frequent interaction between the MRA and the site, which feeds into Merck's goal of building closer relationships with its sites. As a result, the MRA becomes an advocate for the site, and a key link between the site and the in-house team.

As the initiative is rolled out among various studies, Merck will begin measuring its success.

HIPPA and Patient Recruitment

April 14, 2003, was the date by which covered entities were required to comply with the standards of the Privacy Rule under the Health Insurance Portability and Accountability Act of 1996, known as HIPAA. In simple language, the Privacy Rule establishes minimum standards for protecting the privacy of individually identifiable health information. The rule provides individuals with certain rights about how their personal health information (PHI) is used and disclosed, as well as how they can gain access to their health records.

Clinical research is affected by HIPAA regulations as some physicians who conduct clinical studies or administer experimental therapeutics to participants during the course of a study are considered covered entities under HIPAA, meaning that they must comply with the Privacy Rule.

A detailed description of who is or is not considered a covered entity is beyond the scope of this section, but information is available at http://privacyruleandresearch.nih.gov/pr_06.asp#6a. Chapter 3 of this book is dedicated to the subject of HIPAA.

Prospective candidates may find the informed consent process all the more daunting now that it includes the additional HIPAA-related authorization. Savvy investigative sites should consider using this expanded consent process as an opportunity to educate the prospective candidate about specifics of the trial. More interaction between the clinical investigator and the study candidate might be in order to facilitate understanding of what can be a complex set of documents.

This degree of interaction can be an important step toward improving patient retention. If a study subject is in any way confused or overwhelmed by the consent and authorization process, he or she may feel less buy-in to the study, and may be more inclined to drop out. If, however, there is a concerted effort to discuss what will take place during each study visit, and explain the protections offered by the new HIPAA Privacy Rule, the candidate will be more empowered by this knowledge, and may be more inclined to stay in.

Summary: A Look to the Future

The number of clinical trials is on the rise around the globe, and meeting enrollment targets is delayed in most of them due to difficulties in finding qualified volunteers. This is hardly news, but what is new is the degree to which sponsors are embracing professional solutions. Gone are the days in which recruitment is a mere afterthought in the clinical development timeline. Recruitment providers have spent the past decade educating sponsors about the realities of patient recruitment, an activity that is critically important to the success of an investigational compound or device. Clinical professionals need to start thinking about recruitment from the beginning of the protocol development process and then develop tactics specific to various therapeutic indications, accompanied by a budget sufficient to support an appropriate multi-faceted campaign.

Apparently, the educational efforts are working as the recruitment industry is seeing an influx of revenues earmarked for well-designed campaigns dedicated to attracting, recruiting and enrolling study subjects. Current estimates of media spending peg the number at $525 million, a figure that continues to grow. And as the industry becomes more sophisticated, there is a realization that successful patient recruitment is about much more than placing targeted, IRB-approved advertising and counting the number of responses. It is about adding a scientific element to the process by measuring results in a consistent way that leads to the creation of databases of information that will eventually be used to predict success with some degree of certainty. Also, metrics tallied on an ongoing basis enable pro-active changes in media placement throughout the campaign instead of waiting until the end of the study, when it is too late. It is also about the basics…working closely with sites.

As metrics become standard practice, they will eventually be used to measure retention of study subjects, a topic that is gaining increased attention. With one-quarter of volunteers dropping out before study completion, recruitment professionals have set their sights on retention as the next horizon. They have been promoting the idea of treating study subjects as customers who want and expect good customer service. This means convenient hours of operation at the site, being treated with respect, having transportation paid for, getting reminder calls or appointment cards, and being informed about what will happen at each and every study visit. The fact that a recent survey of potential study subjects revealed that prospects were more concerned about an inconvenient trial location than about possibly receiving placebo makes a strong case for the critical importance of good customer service.[18]

New trends are unfolding in patient recruitment and retention. They include increased use of central call centers that do more than field responses to ads. There's also greater use of market research to pinpoint geographic areas with a prevalence of certain diseases, and investigators experienced in treating those conditions. In addition, some market research vendors and sponsors are using focus groups and one-on-one interviews to identify factors that influence willingness to participate in studies, gather opinions on advertising campaigns or gauge perceptions of clinical trials in general.

And finally, there's HIPAA, the set of complex regulations with a Privacy Rule that establishes minimum guidelines for protecting the privacy of individually identifiable health information. While HIPAA has sweeping impact on the healthcare industry at large, it also has the effect of extending the informed consent process because prospective candidates must sign a statement that is either a separate document or attached to the informed consent document explaining their rights under the Privacy Rule. HIPAA also has ramifications for the use of proprietary databases and the selling of lists of names for recruitment purposes.

The increased attention paid to recruitment, enrollment and retention highlights the fact that this aspect of clinical development remains a major issue. This book is dedicated to examining the many dimensions of patient recruitment starting from protocol development, extending to site selection; use of market research to sharpen the focus of multi-media campaigns that use print, radio, television and the Internet; to centralized recruiting; to innovative steps such as sponsors' establishing greater in-house recruitment capability.

Key Takeaways

- With resources pouring into patient recruitment, professional and organized approaches to recruitment and retention are key to meeting or beating enrollment targets and timelines.
- The promise of metrics is that by collecting them routinely, they can populate a database useful in predicting outcomes of recruitment efforts with relative certainty.
- Focusing greater attention on patient retention may serve to reduce the nearly 25% dropout rate of enrolled study volunteers.
- Data suggest that study candidates want to be treated like customers and expect good customer service.
- Sponsors are starting to understand the value of using market research as part of developing multifaceted recruitment campaigns that reach the targeted audience more effectively.
- The Privacy Rule portion of HIPAA, which went into effect for covered entities on April 14, 2003, has a great impact on patient recruitment as study volunteers are to be asked to grant authorization for the use and disclosure of their personal health information (PHI) for a specific study.

References

1. CenterWatch, 2003.
2. Advances in Patient Enrollment, Adherence and Retention in Clinical Trials, DIA meeting, April 2003.
3. CenterWatch surveys of investigative sites, 2003.
4. Rheumatology Research International, 1999.
5. "Improving Recruitment and Retention Practices Based on Input From the Public and Patients," CenterWatch, 2003.
6. CenterWatch, 2003.
7. Op. cit., "Improving Recruitment and Retention Practices Based on Input From the Public and Patients."
8. Ibid., "Improving Recruitment and Retention Practices Based on Input From the Public and Patients."
9. 2003 Assessment of 1700 Pre-Qualified Study Volunteers, Center-Watch, 2003.
10. "Treating Study Volunteers as Customers," *CenterWatch*, Ann Neuer, March 2003, Vol. 10, Issue 3, p. 6.
11. Methods for Improving the Predictability of Clinical Trial Enrollment Rates, Jim Kremidas, DIA Conference, April 29, 2003.
12. "Subject-Focused Performance Drive Clinical Trials," Liz Moench and Beth Harper, *Applied Clinical Trials*, Vol. 6, Number 12, December 1997.
13. Enrollment, Adherence, and Retention: A Broad View, John Needham, DIA Conference, April 29, 2003.
14. Ibid., "Improving Recruitment and Retention Practices Based on Input From the Public and Patients."
15. www.dssresearch.com/library/segment/understanding.asp, accessed May 24, 2003.
16. Ibid., accessed May 25, 2003.
17. Interactive Volunteer Survey, CenterWatch 2002.
18. Ibid.

Author Biography

Diana L. Anderson, Ph.D.
President and CEO, D. L. Anderson International, Inc.

Dr. Diana L. Anderson is the President, CEO and Founder of D. L. Anderson International, Inc., parent company to subsidiaries D. Anderson & Company, a patient recruitment provider and RRI, a Contract Research Organization. D. Anderson & Company, the patient recruitment arm of D. L. Anderson International, Inc., provides a comprehensive menu of specialized services to the clinical trials industry. These services include consulting and patient recruitment management, market research and feasibility assessments, media management and purchasing, creative development, regulatory management, clinical trial branding, community outreach and public relations, site-specific recruitment services, direct-to-consumer strategies, call center support and retention programs.

Dr. Anderson consults globally as a recognized authority in the field of patient recruitment, with recent presentations in Japan, Europe and Israel. She is widely published and frequently featured for her accomplishments in a variety of trade publications and scientific journals. She is also the author of the books *50 Ways to Cope with Arthritis, A Guide to Patient Recruitment* and *A Guide to Patient Recruitment and Retention.*

Dr. Anderson serves on several corporate boards and in various capacities on committees including Immediate Past Chair of the Association of Clinical Research Professionals (ACRP). She has previously held appointments on the Board of Directors of the North Texas Chapter of the Arthritis Foundation; Editorial Board, Arthritis Today Magazine; Past President, Association of Rheumatology Health Professionals (ARHP); Board of Trustees of the National Arthritis Foundation; Board of Directors, American College of Rheumatology; and Past President, Western U.S.A. Pain Society. She maintains memberships and remains actively involved in a number of these professional organizations.

She holds a Ph.D. from Texas Woman's University, M.S.N. from the University of Texas Health Care Science Center in San Antonio, Texas, and a B.S.N. from the University of Nebraska.

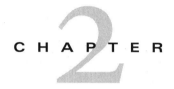

CHAPTER

Benchmarking Patient Recruitment and Retention in Clinical Trials

Kenneth A. Getz

Objectives

- Understand the current climate for patient recruitment and retention.
- Describe four key issues that affect the current patient recruitment climate.
- Identify benchmark descriptive statistics that articulate the size, scope and characteristics of patient recruitment and retention.

Introduction

Every year, several million people participate in clinical trials to support new drug applications (NDAs) submitted to the Food and Drug Administration. This level of participation represents less than 10% of the more than sixty million people who have severe, life-threatening and chronic illnesses in the United States.[1] It would seem relatively easy to find and retain highly motivated study participants from this population for NDA submissions. But that is hardly the case.

At present, the majority (nearly 86%) of clinical trials conducted in the United States fail to enroll subjects within the contract period. This failure rate is up from 80% of trials in the late 1990s.[2] Clearly these delays result in significant direct development costs for the study sponsor. Extended enrollment periods can also cause delays in new product introductions—a substantially higher cost that is due to missed market opportunity. Nearly two-thirds of investigative sites agree that the challenges of patient recruitment and retention are becoming more difficult.[3]

Numbers of Patients Who Volunteer and Enroll in Clinical Trials Annually

Government and industry sponsor more than 80,000 trials in the United States each year, representing as many as 5,000 to 6,000 protocols. The FDA alone reports that there are nearly 4,000 active investigational new drug applications in clinical trials at any one time. An average of sixteen patients is required to complete a protocol, across all therapeutic areas and phases I to III. In total, between 750,000 to 900,000 study subjects will complete clinical trials for new drug applications (NDAs)—many of which will be submitted to the Food and Drug Administration.[4]

The largest numbers of subjects are needed for phase III programs. Seven out of ten study subjects—also called evaluable patients—need to be recruited to support phase III programs for an NDA submission. Slightly less than one in five will be recruited for phase II programs. And 10% of total evaluable patients per NDA will be part of phase I studies.[5]

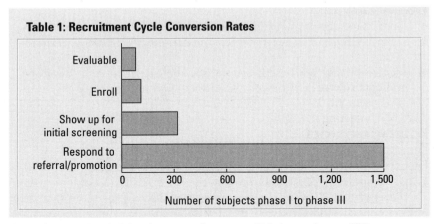

Table 1: Recruitment Cycle Conversion Rates

Source: CenterWatch analysis based on case studies across multiple therapeutic areas, 2002

Most estimates of total study subjects in annual clinical trials fail to capture the much higher numbers of patients that must be drawn into clinical trials in order to yield the required number of subject completions. For example, for every patient who completes a phase I to III clinical trial, three other patients will have an initial screening but will fail to be randomized or then drop out after randomization (see Table 1).

These conversion rates are an aggregation of data from published articles and more than twenty case studies between 1989 and 2002.[6] And, these rates are conservative. Several recent studies suggest that fewer patients are responding to recruitment promotions and fewer still are now completing clinical trials. Using the benchmark conversion rates in Table 1, an estimated 2.8 million to 3.6 million people participate in industry-sponsored clinical trials annually. In other words, each year, several million individuals make a conscious decision, and make the effort, to take part in an initial screening with study staff to determine eligibility.

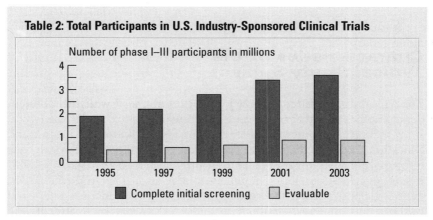

Table 2: Total Participants in U.S. Industry-Sponsored Clinical Trials

Number of phase I–III participants in millions

Complete initial screening   Evaluable

Source: CenterWatch analysis, FDA, PhRMA

These figures represent more than 16,000,000 people who were involved—albeit briefly—in clinical trials in 2003 (see Table 2). This includes those individuals who contacted an investigative site as a result of a professional referral or who responded to a patient recruitment promotion or advertisement. This may reflect some duplication as certain individuals may be contacting investigative sites several times each year to learn about volunteer opportunities. Still, the figures illustrate the challenges of attempting to generate high volumes of potential study subjects in order to yield the required randomized study subject groups.

Overall, these benchmark conversion rates indicate that only one out of every twenty patients who respond to a recruitment promotion ever complete a clinical trial. And, only one out of five patients who respond to a recruitment promotion ever show up for an initial screening.[7]

Estimates of total study subjects participating in industry-sponsored clinical trials do not include phase IV programs. Industry observers speculate that as many as 1.5 to 2 million patients may be involved in pharmacovigilance, periapproval, pharmacoeconomic and registry trials. But this speculation is largely based on anecdotal evidence. At this time there are few to no data published or presented on the number of patients participating nationwide in phase IV programs.

Also, little is known about the number of participants involved in government-funded clinical research. The National Institutes of Health

(NIH) has conducted analyses of specific therapeutic areas including oncology and infectious disease clinical trials. Based on these analyses, the NIH estimates that three to four million patients participate in a wide variety of clinical trials—including biomedical, behavioral and epidemiological programs.[8] The NIH figures also include those individuals who provided informed consent for use of human tissue samples in clinical research studies. The Clinical Research Roundtable, of the Institute of Medicine, recently estimated that 750,000 volunteers completed NIH-funded clinical trials.

Characteristics of the Typical Study Subject

The typical study subject in phase I to III clinical trials has slightly different demographics than that of the general population. In particular, the typical study volunteer is somewhat older and has a lower household income and education level than the general population.[9] Clinical trials are attracting a disproportionate number of older individuals who have a broad range of illnesses targeted by development pipelines today, such as age-related illnesses, neurologic and psychiatric disorders, diseases of the endocrine system and cardiovascular illnesses. Clinical trials that offer free medical treatments and medical care as well as remuneration for participation may be attracting a population in a lower socioeconomic position.

A look at the average U.S. citizen as compared to the average clinical trial participant provides some interesting contrasts. The median age of the U.S. population is thirty-six years. Median household income of the overall U.S. population is $39,600. More than 80% (82%) have at least a high school diploma, and 49% some college education. Almost one out of three (29%) of the overall population has a bachelor's degree or higher. Also, 71% of the general U.S. population is White, 12% is Black, 12% is Hispanic and 4% is Asian.[10]

Based on case studies as well as presentations made by industry analysts and thought leaders, the median age of a clinical trial participant is forty-three years. The median household income for a clinical trial participant is 19% lower—at $33,000—than the national median. And only one out of seven (72%) clinical trial participants has a high school diploma or better, while 38% of study subjects have taken some college classes or have completed college.[11]

Minority Participation on the Rise

Once limited primarily to NIH-funded studies, there has been an unprecedented level of effort to include larger numbers of racial and ethnic minority groups in industry-sponsored clinical trials in the first few years of the 21st century. Several major associations, such as the National Medical Association (the African-American counterpart to the American Medical

Association), the National Alliance for Hispanic Health and the Black Health Network, have implemented formal programs to find and train minority research professionals. Investigative sites and site networks across the United States have emerged with a focus on conducting clinical trials specifically among minority populations.[12]

Historically, FDA guidelines around minority inclusion in clinical trials have been loosely structured. In January 2003, the FDA published draft Guidance for Industry to recommend categories for collecting effectiveness and safety data during clinical trials for ethnic and racial demographic groups. "To accomplish this, FDA recommends that the drug manufacturers use the Office of Management and Budget (OMB) race and ethnicity categories during clinical trial data collection to ensure consistency in evaluating potential differences in drug response among racial and ethnic groups."[13]

There have been observed differences in response to prescribed and investigational drugs in distinct groups of the U.S. population. These differences may be due to genetic makeup, diet, environmental exposure, sociocultural issues or interactions among these factors. For example, in the United States, whites are more likely to have low levels of an important enzyme that metabolizes antidepressants and antipsychotics than people of African or Asian heritage. Other studies have shown that African Americans respond less to several classes of antihypertensive agents (beta blockers and angiotensin converting enzyme [ACE] inhibitors).[14]

A review of new molecular entities (NMEs) approved between 1995 and 1999 reveals that African Americans typically participate in clinical trials at a representative level. Published by the FDA in October 2001, the results indicate that in the United States, African American participation occasionally exceeded proportional prevalence in the overall population. But other minority populations—most notably the Hispanic subgroup—were grossly underrepresented. Only 3% of participants were designated "Hispanic" yet this subgroup comprises 12% of the U.S. population (see Tables 3 and 4).[15]

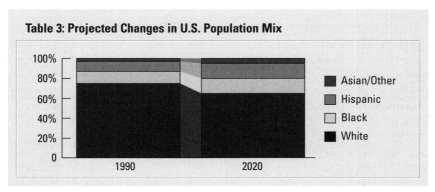

Table 3: Projected Changes in U.S. Population Mix

Source: U.S. Census Bureau, 2000

Table 4: Subgroup Representation in Clinical Trials

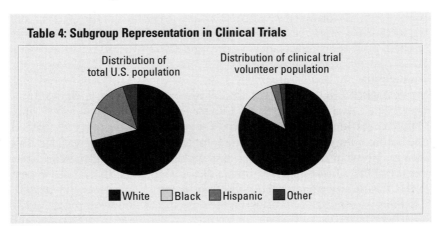

Source: U.S. Census Bureau, 2000

One of the major barriers to trial participation among African Americans is that there is still a general distrust of the medical community—including the pharmaceutical industry and the clinical trial process. The Tuskegee syphilis experiment has contributed greatly to that distrust. In that experiment, researchers actively withheld treatment from hundreds of African American sharecroppers with syphilis. The other major barrier to participation among all minority groups is that only about 7% of the nation's medical doctors belong to a minority group and no more than a handful of them are engaged in clinical research.

Minority patients will often gravitate to physicians of similar race and ethnic background. Thus, some believe that the involvement of minority physicians in the clinical trial has a positive impact on minority recruitment. Educating minority physicians about trials and Good Clinical Practices is the first step toward achieving this goal.[16]

Sponsors are increasingly interested in compiling data on various minority populations and ethnic groups. With the FDA's issuing of its final Guidance for Industry on the Collection of Race and Ethnicity Data in Clinical Trials for FDA-Regulated Products, the interest in including members of minority and ethnic groups is expected to increase in the coming years.[17]

The Inclusion of Women in Clinical Trials

Due to the lack of available data, it has long been believed that the typical study subject is male. Recently gathered data suggest otherwise. It now appears that the gender mix of study volunteers has been distributed equally since 1966.[18] In an October 2000 report published by Controlled Clinical Trials, the authors reviewed 100,000 clinical trials published in reputable journals including the *Lancet*, *NEJM*, *JAMA* and the *Annals of Internal Medicine* between 1966 and 1998. The authors found that 55% of clinical trials involved both men and women, 12% involved men only, and 11% involved women only.

Approximately 21% of the published clinical trials did not specify gender. The authors also noted a higher incidence of male participants involved in cardiovascular studies, a disease that has been long mistakenly believed to affect men disproportionately. And, among cancer trials, women are two-and-a-half times more likely to have been enrolled than are men.

Whereas gender mix in clinical trials appears to be relatively balanced, there is no question that protocol designs have historically addressed disease as it manifests in adult males. During the past decade, public pressures have fueled stricter government requirements for gender-specific studies in both NIH- and industry-sponsored research projects.

Pharmaceutical and biotechnology companies have also sought ways to increase the market potential for new and existing drugs by gathering clinical data to make specific claims about drug safety and effectiveness among women. As a result, clinical trials are increasingly being designed to assess gender-specific medical treatment safety and efficacy.

Many diseases behave differently in women than in men. Risk factors, symptoms, clinical course and response to treatment can all be gender-specific. Among a long list of differences, men and women vary by:

- Body size, composition
- The ways their bodies change during the aging process, e.g., puberty and midlife
- Endogenous hormones
- Exogenous hormones

Although the FDA recommended in 1993 that clinical studies include enough women to understand the unique ways in which their bodies respond to drugs, more than a decade later, women are still underrepresented in small phase I safety trials. And when eligibility is restricted by age, older women are disproportionately excluded from studies of diseases that are more common in women at older ages. The possibility of becoming pregnant also excludes most women in their childbearing years.[19]

Generally a woman capable of conceiving a child won't be considered for a clinical trial unless she's not pregnant and agrees to use birth control. Many studies require that women of childbearing age use two forms of contraception during participation. Pharmaceutical companies don't want their drugs tested among women who are—or might get—pregnant, mostly because the risk of a lawsuit by the mother is too high. Many parents are quick to blame poor birth outcomes on drugs. Some doctors erroneously believe that certain drugs cause fetal abnormalities. But genes and chromosomes are the primary culprits, according to Marilynn C. Frederiksen, M.D., associate professor of obstetrics and gynecology at Northwestern University Medical School.[20]

All of this presents a major barrier to clinical trial participation by women who don't want, can't afford or are religiously opposed to contraception. Things aren't bound to change unless the National Institutes of Health (NIH) comes up with the funds to conduct special dosing studies in pregnant women, said Frederiksen. And that probably won't happen quickly or easily. The NIH doesn't have any institutes that devote research dollars specifically to women's health issues.[21]

As a direct result of the 1993 NIH Revitalization Act, NIH-sponsored clinical research now routinely includes sufficient numbers of non-pregnant women. Pharmaceutical companies following FDA guidelines, however, pay for most clinical trials. The FDA recommended in 1977 that premenopausal women capable of becoming pregnant be excluded from early drug trials. In practice, the participation of women in all phases was affected. The FDA's current stance—that a "reasonable" number of women be included in all clinical trials—hasn't fully addressed participation inequities.[22]

In trials where women are included, the Government Accounting Office recently reported that about one-third of pharmaceutical companies fail to present gender-specific safety and efficacy data in their new drug application (NDA) summaries, as required by the FDA. NDAs also frequently arrive at the FDA without any recommended dose adjustments based on sex. Similarly, investigational new drug annual reports routinely leave out the number of study participants by gender.[23]

The participation of women in clinical trials is essential. Real-world experience has proven that some drugs that work well in men may be ineffective or more dangerous in women, regardless of body size. Pharmaceutical companies are devoting a tremendous amount of money to trials focusing on diseases and conditions that only affect women. They're also pushing for more representative patient populations in their non-sex-specific studies. But women can be a challenge to recruit for trials because the protocols written for them tend to involve a lot of time-consuming tests.[24]

Pediatric Clinical Trials

Since children have been excluded from clinical trials historically, many of the drugs that are now prescribed to children have never been tested on that population during the drug development process. Recent and pending legislation, such as the Pediatric Rule and the proposed Pediatric Research Act of 2003, are dedicated to making pediatric clinical trials into an integral part of drug development—which, in turn, translates into greater demand and competition for pediatric trial subjects. It also brings into high relief the concerns over adequate protection of pediatric subjects. One such concern is about compensation for child subjects' participation as a motivating factor.[25]

But there is encouraging news according to a Pediatric Clinical Trials International survey conducted recently of 132 respondents (74 parents and 58 subjects age 9 or older) who represented participants enrolled in 21 industry-sponsored phase I-IV studies. Sixty-nine percent of subjects and 72% of parents described the level of care that the child received from the doctor/staff as "much better than expected." In addition, 49% of subjects responded that they would "definitely consider" participating in another study, and 76% of parents responded that they would "definitely consider" having their child participate in another clinical trial.[26]

Most parents hear about a clinical trial through their physician. Thus, trust in that physician is of paramount importance. The reputation of the participating institution also plays an important role. Most parents respond quickly to an effective, targeted media campaign for a pediatric trial, so advertising tactics can be quickly assessed.[27]

Common Characteristics of Study Subjects

Study subjects are uniquely motivated to find and access new medical treatments. Of the three million people who participate in clinical trials in the United States each year, an estimated 40% receive their primary care from a staff-model HMO or managed care provider. More than 70% of the U.S. population receives its primary care through a managed care network.[28] Still, study volunteers are expressing a high motivation level as they are stepping outside their health care network, often without the permission of their primary care physician or nurse.

There has been a dramatic shift in study participant self-referral behavior. In a survey conducted among several hundred patients in 1995, only one-third of patients said that they self-referred into a clinical trial. Their physician or nurse referred them to a clinical trial nearly two-thirds of the time. In 2004, 50% of patients said they self-refer into a clinical trial and 34% said that their physician or nurse had referred them. And in surveys among several thousand health consumers, 60% of consumers say they would be willing to participate in an appropriate clinical trial, despite the fact that most patients (74%) claim that they know little to nothing about the clinical research process and what is expected of them.[29] A poll of 5,348 adults conducted in May 2003 finds that 77% of consumers would consider participating in a clinical research study if their physician asked them to.[30]

Clinical research coordinators, clinical investigators and study staff strongly agree that today's patients are more informed about their medical conditions and their treatment options. Driven in large part by healthcare reform during the past decade, patients are less trusting of a single medical opinion. And patients and their advocates want to take more responsibility for their treatment decisions. However, motivation to seek out information about treatment options has not extended rapidly into the clinical research arena. With the exception of those patients with the most severe and life-threatening illnesses, most people do not readily consider clinical research a treatment option. And their providers of primary and specialized health services—again with the exception of severe, life-threatening illnesses—typically do not suggest or recommend clinical trial participation.

In a survey conducted in 2000 among 1,000 people, 77% said they have never spoken with their physician or nurse about participating in clinical trials.[31] Only one in five patients (22%) have. These findings suggest a major opportunity for the NIH and industry to educate patients, the general public and health professionals on the value and the risks and benefits of clinical research participation.

How Potential Study Participants Identify Clinical Trial Opportunities

Investigative sites have traditionally turned to the following approaches in order to identify potential study subjects: Chart review, walk-ins, professional referrals, phone screens, study notices and bulletins and direct mail to patients and physician practices. During the past decade, investigative sites have also dramatically increased their use of the mass media to reach prospective volunteers, newspaper ads, radio advertising, television and more recently, the Internet. These strategies, and the ways in which they are affected by compliance with the Health Insurance Portability and Accountability Act [HIPAA] Privacy Rule, are covered in depth throughout this book.

Interestingly, recruitment approaches vary by investigative site type. And, the recruitment approaches used by investigative sites have a direct impact on the type of volunteer enrolled in clinical trials (see Table 5). Traditional investigative sites (i.e., major medical centers and part-time sites) rely more heavily on their own patients or on physician referral. More than 70% of major medical centers, for example, say that their study subjects come from internal sources, including physician faculty and affiliated physician networks.

Part-time sites, investigative sites that derive revenue from both clinical practice and clinical trials, report a mix of approaches that favor the patient community that they directly serve. These traditional study conduct

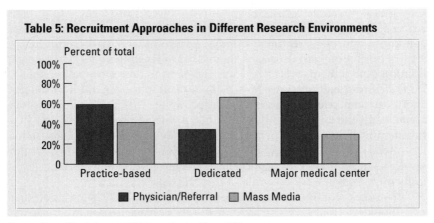

Table 5: Recruitment Approaches in Different Research Environments

Source: CenterWatch Survey of 103 Investigative Sites, 1999

providers tend to attract a larger percentage of patients from actual use settings where patients are seen and treated by their primary care or specialty care providers.

Dedicated investigative sites, including many that are site management organizations, are research center sites that derive almost 100% of their revenue from clinical trial activities—relying heavily on mass media advertising and promotion to find study subjects. Certain dedicated sites maintain a full-time staff of principal investigators and study coordinators. In these instances, study volunteers are often seen only during a clinical trial and not in an actual use setting.

Ultimately, the variability in patient recruitment approaches across investigative site environments raises issues about where sponsors and CROs should place their clinical trials and the number of dollars that should be budgeted for patient recruitment approaches. This variability in recruitment behavior across investigative site types extends beyond the United States. The use of mass media for patient recruitment is growing in parts of Europe as well.[32]

Today, patients still prefer to gather their general health and medical information from their physician or nurse. In a survey of 1,565 people in the United States:

- 58% of respondents said they turn to their doctor or nurse for health information;
- 39% refer to the newspaper or other mass media for health-related information;
- 28% learn about trials through flyers posted at the research center
- 14% respondents browse the Internet for this information[33]

In the same survey, the vast majority of people (85%) felt that it is very important that their doctor or nurse get involved or refer them to a clinical research program. Yet, as mentioned earlier, only a small percentage of the general public reports that their doctor or nurse ever mentions clinical trials as a treatment consideration.

The above statistics touch on sources for general health information. Another recent survey looked specifically at where patients learn about clinical trials.[34] These data are skewed toward individuals who completed a clinical trial within the past year:

- Almost half of study subjects (46%) said that a physician or nurse actually referred them to the trial;
- One-third (35%) of study volunteers said they learned about a trial through mass media venues—newspapers, TV, radio, magazines and press releases;
- Fewer than one in ten study subjects reported that they first learned of a clinical trial through the Internet; and
- Approximately 2% of study subjects reported that they learned of a clinical trial through cold calls that originated from a research center.

When an individual learns about a clinical trial, he or she is most likely to call the research center by telephone, with 70% choosing to do so. One in five (19%) prefers to show up at a research center in person. At present, 10% prefer to contact a center by email.[35]

Motivators of Clinical Trial Participation

Based on a survey of more than 1,200 study volunteers who had completed phase II and III clinical trials within the past year, the largest percentage of study subjects gets involved to find a more effective treatment.[36] Approximately one in four study volunteers gets involved for altruistic reasons—they hope to advance science. Only 11% of study subjects say they become involved primarily to earn extra money. And fewer than one in ten (6%) volunteers to participate in order to receive better medical care and for help covering the cost of therapy. These findings are consistent with the results of similar surveys conducted in the early 1990s.

A high percentage—61%—of the general public say that they would likely get involved in a clinical trial. However, in a recent Harris Interactive poll of several thousand Americans, of patients who are aware of a suitable clinical trial, most, 71%, choose not to participate.[37]

There are similar results with Internet-based listings of clinical trials. At present, only an estimated 34% of individuals follow up with investigative sites when they find an appropriate clinical trial listing on the CenterWatch web site. In a recent survey, the top reasons why people choose not to participate have to do with fears about experiencing side effects and dealing with participation-related inconveniences (see Table 6). Fear of receiving a placebo instead of the active drug is also a major factor reducing patient willingness to volunteer.[38]

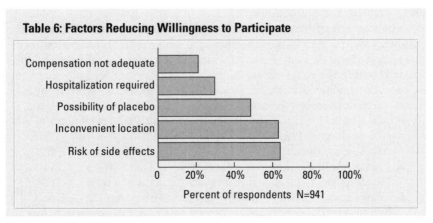

Table 6: Factors Reducing Willingness to Participate

Percent of respondents N=941

Source: CenterWatch, 2002

The Impact of Poor Recruitment and Retention

Prospective volunteer management initiatives may very well be some of the largest determinants of volunteer willingness to participate in a clinical trial. Forty percent of pre-qualified patients fail to enroll in clinical trials due to inconvenience and poor customer service. In a survey of more than 1,700 pre-qualified study volunteers for phase II and III projects, 13% never enrolled because there was no conveniently located investigative site. Fourteen percent of pre-qualified patients lost interest following their initial interactions with a call center or study staff. And, 23% of pre-qualified volunteers were never randomized because no one contacted them after the initial phone screen.[39]

A separate study of nearly 1,000 patients corroborates these findings. In that survey, research center location and hours of operation are two of the top factors influencing volunteers' decisions to participate. For survey respondents, these factors ranked substantially higher than concerns about the possibility of receiving placebo. In fact, the results of this survey suggest that convenience is a large concern to volunteers as is the fear of side effects from the investigational drug.[40]

In the survey of 1,700 patients, respondents reported that not having enough information about the trial was one of the top five reasons for not participating in the study. Patients appear to be eager to understand more about the required number of visits and the logistics of their participation. Responsiveness to volunteer inquiries and volunteer interest can have a dramatic impact on recruitment.[41]

And an analysis of IRB completion records of more than 25,000 study subjects conducted in 2003 shows that volunteer retention rates are much lower than originally expected. In this analysis, only 73% of enrolled volunteers completed their clinical trials—26% dropped out. Moreover, there is considerable variability in retention rates across clinical trial phases. Volunteer retention rates are the lowest in phase II/III studies and highest in phase IV programs.[42]

Clinical research professionals say that there are a numerous reasons why volunteers drop out of trials. Some of the most common include lack of efficacy, adverse reactions, excessive study duration, too large a commitment required from volunteers and invasive procedures. Although many causes of volunteer dropout cannot be prevented, most investigative sites believe that much can be done to improve retention rates through more effective and continuous management of the investigative site-subject relationship beginning with initial interactions through randomization and eventual study completion.

Given that enrollment and retention failures are the largest causes of overall delays in drug development, it is critical that sponsors, CROs and sites apply principles of excellent customer service into the overall recruitment and retention process. Customer-oriented clinical research professionals are finding that convenient center locations and hours, ease of scheduling appointments, prompt return of phone calls, good parking arrangements, customer-friendly protocols—even good listening skills—offer major advantages to study conduct performance.[43]

Building and implementing customer service initiatives require broad support from project managers through to investigative site personnel. Protocol design, for example, may be patient-unfriendly—requiring too many visits, visits that are too long or that include invasive and unpleasant procedures. By the same token, underenrolling sites may lack the infrastructure or operational support to provide the level of customer service required. Phone coverage may be weak or supported by a poorly trained staff member. Volunteers may never feel fully connected or valued by the research center.[44]

Some investigative sites and sponsors are making strides in providing higher levels of customer service, but most industry professionals argue that there is still a long way to go. Many sites are overburdened and short-staffed. They cannot provide the level of customer service that sponsors believe would effectively deliver recruitment and retention goals. Similarly, most investigative site personnel find that sponsors don't understand the challenges of providing quality customer service under the constraints presented by the protocol.[45]

Ideally, over time, improvements in customer satisfaction hold the promise of reducing industry focus on casting a wide net in order to reach and attract as many new potential candidates as possible. Indeed, across industries a major tenet of effective customer service is the recognition that new customer acquisition is far more expensive than that of keeping existing customers. Satisfying volunteers already in clinical trials—treating them as valued and loyal customers—is a primary means of better addressing that rising costs and development cycle delays caused by poor patient recruitment and retention.[46]

Industry Spending to Facilitate Patient Recruitment

It is estimated that, combined, sponsors, CROs and sites spent $445 million in 2003 on patient recruitment promotional activities. This represents less than 2% of total clinical development spending.[47]

Based on surveys of several hundred investigative sites, an estimated $250 million is directly allocated by the investigative sites for the purposes of patient recruitment.[48] This figure does not include the costs of routine personnel and overhead. This figure represents spending for marketing programs—typically local promotional programs including flyers, outreach initiatives, mailings and limited mass media activities. Investigative sites report that they spend approximately 6% of every study grant on patient recruitment promotion.[49]

While it is true that sponsors are paying larger than average grants-per-study to investigative sites, increased grant spending is not the result of rising costs-per-patient. Cost-per-patient has risen less than 5% annually from approximately $4,500 in fees-per-patient in 1990 to $6,700 in 2002. When adjusted for inflation, the cost-per-patient has been essentially flat. This suggests that investigative sites are conducting a growing number of procedures per patient for less average funding per procedure.[50]

The amount paid to investigative sites, when adjusted for inflation, is hardly rising, meaning that at the same time that recruitment is becoming more difficult, sites are doing more with less. Study costs are rising because more procedures are being performed on each study volunteer. This factor is contributing to increased difficulty in study subject compliance and retention.

Pharmaceutical and CRO companies spend an additional $175 to $200 million directly on mass media patient recruitment promotions for phase I to III programs.[51] Much of this spending is allocated to advertising agencies to cover large regional and national campaigns to support patient recruitment programs. A portion of sponsor and CRO spending may also be going to investigative sites as remedial support. As a result, sponsors and CRO spending on patient recruitment may include some duplication of investigative site spending.

The vast majority (93%) of investigative sites report that they rely on their study coordinator(s) for most patient recruitment responsibilities. Yet study coordinators, busy running most daily research study activities, are typically not trained to manage large marketing and promotional programs. Fewer than one in three (28%) investigative sites report that they depend on administrative support to direct patient recruitment initiatives.[52] Only 13% of investigative sites report having a dedicated patient recruitment specialist. This is an interesting and concerning fact given that investigative sites and sponsors strongly agree that patient enrollment rates are the single largest determinant of repeat business.

Summary

Clinical projects are more ambitious today than ever before. Several seminal studies have been recently published that document the rising number of clinical studies per new drug application (NDA), the growth in the number of procedures performed per protocol and the increasing numbers of study subjects required per NDA.

Drug pipelines are also growing at a faster rate given the impact of new drug discovery technologies including high throughput screening, combinatorial chemistry, and pharmacogenomics. In 1993, there were an estimated 4,000 projects in the drug development pipeline. In 2003, that number has more than doubled.[54] The number of new drugs entering this pipeline is projected to grow by 12% annually during the next five years.

This is almost twice the growth rate of new drugs entering the pipeline during the past five years.

There is significant pressure on pharmaceutical companies to increase their development productivity and to improve the performance of drugs once they enter the market. Industry observers expect sponsor companies to invest far more heavily in the coming years to improve the patient recruitment process during clinical development in order to gather more data about investigational treatments and to prime the market, to engage more physician prescribers, prior to product launch. The patient recruitment process has historically been the largest single cause of delays in clinical development.

A number of factors cause recruitment difficulties. For example, protocols may be too stringent, resulting in eligibility requirements that exclude too many. Protocols may be too demanding. And as a result, patient volunteers are asked to contribute more than is reasonable to subject themselves to unpleasant and invasive procedures. There may be too many trials competing for the same patients. Or, clinical trials may be competing with medical therapies that, although not ideal, are effective enough to diminish interest in accessing a therapy that is only available through clinical trial participation. Lastly, potential study subjects may associate a high level of risk with participating in clinical trials. To date, NIH and industry have not effectively educated the general public about the importance of clinical research. Doing so would benefit all parties involved in the clinical trial process—patients, health professionals and clinical research professionals.

Several process and technology changes are addressing some of the difficulties described above. As a result, we may eventually see a decline in the number of evaluable patients per NDA; a decrease in the number of procedures per clinical trial; and a decline in the number of studies per NDA.

Over time, electronic data management technologies may make it easier to target specific patient populations. Electronic data management technologies may also arm study sponsors and staff with real-time abilities to monitor and improve clinical trial performance. The Internet may become a more viable distribution channel to reach potential study subjects. And this approach may offer cost advantages over other mass media approaches.

Pharmacogenomic research and studies for special populations (e.g., pediatrics, minorities and gender-specific) may drive smaller clinical trials in which far more targeted and select patients will be recruited. Sponsor companies are also committing resources and attention to developing protocols and project plans that are more targeted to real-world patient populations. These approaches may result in more inclusive eligibility criteria.

Investigative sites are forming larger and broader networks that include a variety of health providers, including tertiary care and community-based physicians, private-payor and managed care settings, and multi-specialty and population-specialty environments.

These are but a few of the changes in clinical development practices that may have profound effects on the patient recruitment process in the coming decade. Understanding of the process today combined with the application of exciting solutions to address process improvement areas will no doubt facilitate the use of more effective strategies and practices in the new frontiers of patient recruitment.

The data presented in this chapter provide benchmark characteristics of the current climate for patient recruitment and retention. The insights gleaned from these data suggest numerous opportunities for research sponsors, CROs, service providers and investigative sites to collectively improve patient recruitment and retention effectiveness.

Key Takeaways

- More than 2.5 million people complete clinical trials in the United States each year. This represents approximately 10% of the population eligible that participates in clinical trials One out of every four randomized volunteers drops out of a clinical trial every year. These statistics suggest a large opportunity to improve trial recruitment and retention effectiveness.
- Study volunteers are motivated to participate in clinical research for a wide variety of reasons. This complex combination of motivations ranges from wanting to help in the advancement of science, to seeking a better medical therapy, to finding an accessible and convenient volunteer experience.
- Most study volunteers self-refer into clinical trials that were identified through mass media promotions (e.g., newspaper, radio and television). Only one out of four volunteers reports learning about clinical trials through their primary and specialty care providers.
- There is a valuable major opportunity to provide early public and patient-oriented education about the clinical research enterprise. A high percentage of the general public say that they would like to get involved in a clinical trial, though most report having limited to no knowledge about clinical trials and the drug development process. Following their completion of clinical trials, the vast majority of volunteers say that they would participate again.

References

1. U.S. Census Bureau, Statistical Abstract of the United States, August 2000.
2. Getz, K. "Meeting and Extending Enrollment Deadlines." PAREXEL Pharmaceutical R&D Statistical Sourcebook 2000. Page 104.

3. Zisson, S. "Losing Ground in the Battle Against Development Delays." *CenterWatch Newsletter*, 1998. Vol. 5. Issue 12. Pages 1, 3-6.
4. CenterWatch Editors. "Grant Market to Exceed $4 Billion in 2000." *CenterWatch Newsletter*, 2000. Vol. 7. Issue 11. Pages 1, 6-10.
5. Ibid.
6. Ibid.

Lovato, et al. "Recruitment for Controlled Clinical Trials Literature Summary." *Controlled Clinical Trials*, 1997. Vol. 18. Pages 328-357.

Silagy, C.A., et al. "Comparison of Recruitment Strategies for Large Scale Clinical Trials in the Elderly." *Journal of Clinical Epidemiology*, 1991. Vol. 44. Pages 1105-1114.

Spilker, B. and Cramer J. *Patient Recruitment in Clinical Trials*. Raven Press, 1992. Pages 39-59.

Swinehart, J.M. "Patient Recruitment and Enrollment in Clinical Trials: A Discussion of Specific Methods and Disease States." *Journal of Clinical Research and Pharmacoepidemiology*, 1991. Vol. 5. Pages 35-47.

Yusuf, S., et al. "Selection of Patients for Randomized Controlled Trials: Implications of Wide or Narrow Eligibility Criteria." *Statistics in Medicine*, 1990. Vol. 9. Pages 73-83.

Comis, R. "Harris Poll Data on Public and Patient Views of the National Cancer Clinical Trials." Presented at the Institute of Medicine's Clinical Research Roundtable, Washington, DC, September 25, 2000.

Getz, K. "Study Volunteer Behaviors and Attitudes in Industry-Sponsored Clinical Trials." Presented at the Institute of Medicine's Clinical Research Roundtable, Washington, DC, September 25, 2000.

7. Ibid.
8. Comis, R. "Harris Poll Data on Public and Patient Views of the National Cancer Clinical Trials." Presented at the Institute of Medicine's Clinical Research Roundtable, Washington DC, September 25, 2000.
9. CenterWatch Editors. "A Word from Clinical Trials Volunteers." *CenterWatch* 1999. Vol. 6, Issue 6. Pages 1, 9-13.
10. U.S. Census Bureau, Statistical Abstract of the United States, August 2000.
11. Lovato, et al. "Recruitment for Controlled Clinical Trials Literature Summary." *Controlled Clinical Trials*, 1997. Vol. 18. Pages 328-357.
12. Borfitz, Deborah. "Improving Minority Inclusion," *CenterWatch* 2002 Vol. 9, Issue 2, pp. 1, 8-12.
13. FDA Guidance for Industry: Collection of Race and Ethnicity Data in Clinical Trials. January 2003.
14. Ibid.
15. Borfitz, Deborah. "Improving Minority Inclusion," *CenterWatch* 2002 Vol. 9, Issue 2, pp. 1, 8-12.
16. Ibid.
17. Ibid.

18. Meinert, C. "Study Finds Women Not Under-Represented in U.S. Clinical Trials." *Controlled Clinical Trials*, October 2000.
19. Getz, Kenneth A.; Borfitz, Deborah. *Informed Consent: The Guide to the Risks and Benefits of Volunteering for Clinical Trials*, CenterWatch 2002.
20. Ibid.
21. Ibid.
22. Ibid.
23. Ibid.
24. Ibid.
25. Niles, John P., "Pediatric Subjects and Their Parents" *Applied Clinical Trials* 2003, Vol. 12, No. 4.
26. Ibid.
27. Ibid.
28. Getz, K. "Improving Recruitment and Retention in Industry-Sponsored Clinical Trials." Presented at the Drug Information Association Meeting, April, 2003.
29. Ibid.
30. Harris Interactive, "The Many Reasons Why People Participate in Clinical Trials." June 2003 Healthcare Newsletter.
31. Woolley, M. "Research!America Poll Data on Attitudes Toward Medical Research." Presented at the Institute of Medicine's Clinical Research Roundtable, Washington DC, September 25, 2000.
32. Gambrill, Sara. "National Recruitment Programs in Europe Making Inroads." *CenterWatch* 2002, Vol. 9, Issue 8.
33. CenterWatch 2002 Survey.
34. Getz, K. "Study Volunteer Behaviors and Attitudes in Industry-Sponsored Clinical Trials." Presented at the Institute of Medicine's Clinical Research Roundtable, Washington, DC, September 25, 2000.
35. Ibid.
36. Ibid.
37. Woolley, M. "Research!America Poll Data on Attitudes Toward Medical Research." Presented at the Institute of Medicine's Clinical Research Roundtable, Washington, DC, September 25, 2000.
38. Getz, Kenneth A. "Improving Recruitment and Retention in Industry-Sponsored Clinical Trials." Presented at the Drug Information Association meeting, April 2003, based on CenterWatch survey of 970 prospective volunteers.
39. Neuer, Ann. "Treating Study Volunteers as Customers" *CenterWatch* 2003, Vol. 10, Issue 3.
40. Ibid.
41. Ibid.
42. Gamache, Valerie. "Minimizing Volunteer Dropout" *CenterWatch* 2002, Vol. 9, Issue 12.
43. Ibid.
44. Ibid.
45. Ibid.

46. Ibid.
47. Getz, K. "Improving Recruitment and Retention in Industry-Sponsored Clinical Trials." Presented at the Drug Information Association Meeting, April 2003.
48. Henderson, Lisa, et al. "Sites Prosper...But Financial Health Threatened." *CenterWatch*, 2000. Vol. 7, Issue 1. Pages 1, 10-14.
49. Ibid.
50. DataEdge, CenterWatch analysis.
51. Getz, K. "Study Volunteer Behaviors and Attitudes in Industry-Sponsored Clinical Trials." Presented at the Institute of Medicine's Clinical Research Roundtable, Washington, DC.
52. CenterWatch Editors. "Clinical Grants Market Decelerates" *CenterWatch* 2003 Vol. 10, Issue 4. Pages 1, 6-10.

Author Biography

Kenneth A. Getz
Former president and founder of CenterWatch

Mr. Getz is a speaker at industry conferences and has published articles and chapters in a variety of journals and books. He is also the co-author of a book for patients and their advocates entitled *Informed Consent: A Guide to the Risks and Benefits of Volunteering for Clinical Trials*. Mr. Getz has appeared on radio and television programs to speak with patients and their advocates about the clinical trial process.

He holds an MBA from the J.L. Kellogg Graduate School of Management at Northwestern University and a bachelor's degree, Phi Beta Kappa, from Brandeis University.

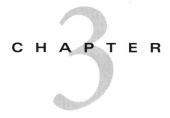

CHAPTER 3

The HIPAA Privacy Rule's Impact on Patient Recruitment

Ellen Kelso Holt and Sheila Elliott Kinney, J.D.

Objectives

- Identify areas where the HIPAA Privacy Rule will have an impact on recruiting efforts.
- Understand how to use protected health information for patient recruitment under the HIPAA Privacy Rule.

Introduction

Both government and industry are trying to increase public awareness of clinical trials and trust in the clinical trial process through the targeted, strategic dissemination of information. The comprehensive registry of all clinical trials for serious illness mandated by Congress in 2000 and the proliferation of web sites providing information about the clinical trials process and the ability for patients to self-refer are examples of these efforts.

Traditionally, recruitment and retention efforts have been dependent on individual investigative site efforts to develop and place advertisements, pre-screen callers, manage patient databases, schedule appointments, provide appointment reminders and other services that help patients attend study visits. These methods depend exclusively on research sites and their resources for successful recruitment and retention. The increasing challenges are motivating new strategies involving centrally orchestrated recruitment campaigns and retention services.

To positively impact the enrollment of patients for clinical trials, marketing or advertising agencies specializing in patient recruitment are blending advertising with public relations and other novel marketing initiatives, including the Internet. This current trend shifts the patient recruitment focus from the individual investigator to centralized patient recruitment campaigns.

This chapter will discuss the basics of the HIPAA Privacy Rule (Privacy Rule), its impact on the recruitment of patients as clinical research subjects and will provide guidance on the current methods for recruiting and retaining patients under the Privacy Rule.

HIPAA Privacy Rule "Personal Health Information" (PHI)

The Privacy Rule's regulations apply to "personal health information" (PHI), which is (1) "health information" that is (2) "individually identifiable" and is (3) created or received by a "covered entity." Health information is "individually identifiable" under HIPAA if it directly identifies an individual or could be used to identify an individual. Health information directly identifies an individual if it includes any of eighteen (18) direct identifiers specified by HIPAA (see Table 1).

Items 1-17 in Table 1 describe demographic information that directly identifies an individual ("direct identifiers"). Item 18 is a catchall category that covers any identifier that HIPAA did not specify in Items 1-17 that could be used to identify an individual. Importantly Item 18 includes an "identifying code." Under HIPAA, an identifying code is one that is derived in some way from the data set or an individual's identification. An example would be the last four digits of a person's social security number. Such a code is an "indirect identifier" that renders the data set "identifiable" because the code could possibly be used to re-identify the individual. In contrast, a nonidentifying code is one that is not derived from the data and could not feasibly be used to re-identify the individual.

In summary, individually identifiable health information (IIHI) has two components: health information and identifying demographic information. The latter could include direct identifiers (Items 1-17 in Table 1) and/or an indirect identifier (an identifying code, Item 18 in Table 1).

HIPAA Privacy Rule: The Basics

The most significant impact of the HIPAA Privacy Rule for investigators is in the area of patient recruitment. In an update to the Privacy Rule, effective August 14, 2002, the HHS clarified that recruitment of subjects for research is indeed "research." Therefore, common recruitment practices such as records review and use of databases are now subject to the restrictions imposed by the Privacy Rule.

Table 1: HIPAA Identifiers

1. Names (initials do not have to be removed);

2. All geographic subdivisions smaller than a State, including ZIP Code (except for the first 3 digits of the ZIP Code if the region contains > 20,000 people, or the last 2 digits if the region contains ≤ 20,000 people);

3. All elements of dates (except year), including birth, death, admission and discharge dates; all ages over 89 years (may include age ≤ 89 years)

4. Telephone numbers;

5. Fax numbers;

6. Electronic mail addresses;

7. Social security numbers;

8. Medical record numbers;

9. Health plan beneficiary numbers;

10. Account numbers;

11. Certificate/license numbers;

12. Vehicle identifiers and serial numbers, including license plate numbers;

13. Device identifiers and serial numbers;

14. Universal Resource Locators (URLs);

15. Internet Protocol (IP) address numbers

16. Biometric identifiers, including finger and voice prints;

17. Full face photographic images and any comparable images; and

18. Any other unique identifying number, characteristic or code.

The Privacy Rule establishes the conditions under which protected health information (PHI) may be used or disclosed by covered entities for any purpose, including research. Covered entities include health plans and health care clearinghouses, and health care providers that electronically transmit PHI. Not every healthcare provider is a covered entity; but, for those that are, the Privacy Rule governs the use and disclosure of PHI that is transmitted or maintained in any form—electronic, paper or oral. This discussion assumes that investigators conducting research are covered entities under the Privacy Rule.

The Privacy Rule requires that a covered entity:

- Provide individuals prior notice of its policy (Privacy Notice) regarding the way that entity may use or disclose PHI,
- Describe what its responsibilities are with respect to such information, and
- Describe the rights individuals have and how they may exercise them.

A covered entity's practices must be consistent with those described in the Privacy Notice and any use and disclosure of PHI should be limited to the minimum necessary to achieve the purpose intended.

The Privacy Rule also requires a covered entity to enter into a written contract (Business Associate Contract) with persons or businesses performing certain covered functions on their behalf that involve PHI. The covered functions define the PHI that can be used or disclosed without patient permission for the purpose of providing individual treatment, to facilitate insurance payments and to measure and improve performance of those two activities.

The Privacy Rule specifies that a covered entity may not use or disclose PHI for research purposes unless the subject has provided, in advance, his/her written authorization (Authorization) for such use or disclosure. Under the Privacy Rule, an Authorization allows simply for the use and disclosure of PHI for research purposes.

The Privacy Rule supplements federal human research policies by requiring that the protection of confidentiality in research be handled in a very specific way. Research funded by states or private sponsors is not regulated by federal human research policies. The Privacy Rule is broader than federal human research policies in that it extends to all research, regardless of funding, and to both living and deceased individuals.

Where the Privacy Rule and federal human research policies are applicable, both must be followed. Where they overlap, the most stringent standard applies. Similarly, state law continues to apply where it is more restrictive than the Privacy Rule.

Obtaining Authorization

The form used to obtain valid Authorization is specified in the Privacy Rule. Individuals must be provided, in writing, the relevant information on which to base their decision to allow the uses/disclosures of PHI.

Six essential elements apply to an Authorization regardless of the purpose for the use or disclosure:

1. A description of what information will be used
2. Who will use it

3. To whom it will be disclosed
4. For what purpose
5. The expiration date
6. The patient's dated signature

The Authorization must also provide notice of a patient's right to revoke the Authorization, the ability of the investigator to condition research participation on the Authorization and of the potential for PHI to be re-disclosed.

An Authorization must be specific in the description of these elements and notices and investigators should take care to identify and include any secondary uses and disclosures (re-disclosures) that might be associated with the research, e.g., disclosures to sub-investigators not within the investigator's covered entity or to organizations providing participant retention or communication services. The expiration date for research Authorizations may be indicated as "end of the study" (or "none" for an Authorization to place PHI in a research database).

The Privacy Rule does not require review and approval of (stand-alone) Authorization forms prior to use. However, the covered entity is accountable for compliance with these requirements and may require an internal approval procedure (by a forms committee, HIPAA compliance board or their IRB). To enroll research subjects, investigators must obtain signatures on both the Authorization and the informed consent document required by federal human research policies. The regulations allow the two to be combined into one document. But in some cases, the requirement for an Authorization may be triggered separately or prior to the requirement for informed consent. For instance, HIPAA Authorization is required to disclose PHI already in existence to an investigator, who is not part of the covered entity, for the purpose of identifying potential research subjects.

Revocation—the Reliance Exception

Upon receipt of written revocation, the covered entity must stop using/disclosing PHI, except to the extent that the covered entity has acted in reliance on the Authorization. For research, the reliance exception would permit the continued use and disclosure of PHI to account for subjects' withdrawal from the research study, to include in safety or efficacy analyses for a marketing application submitted to the FDA, to conduct any investigation of misconduct or to report adverse events. However, information gathered after revocation may not be used or disclosed, even under the reliance exception.

Other Ways to Obtain PHI for Research Purposes

Short of a HIPAA Authorization, there are several ways PHI may be obtained for research. Covered entities may obtain documentation that an IRB or Privacy Board has granted a waiver of the required Authorization (Waiver). Covered entities may also use PHI without Authorization if a researcher represents that the PHI is necessary to prepare for research or that the PHI is solely for research on decedents.

Waiver of Authorization

Protected health information used or disclosed under a Waiver is subject to the minimum necessary standard. To grant a Waiver, an IRB or Privacy Board must find that the research satisfies the following criteria:
1. There is "minimal risk to privacy" which includes meeting three criteria:
   a. There is an adequate plan to protect patient identifiers;
   b. There is an adequate plan to destroy identifiers at the earliest opportunity (unless there is a health or research justification or it is required by law); and
   c. There are adequate written assurances against re-disclosure.
2. The research could not be practicably conducted without the Waiver.
3. The research could not be practicably conducted without access to PHI.

Before use or disclosure is permitted, covered entities must receive documentation of the Waiver that includes: the identity of the IRB or Privacy Board and Waiver approval date, a brief description of the PHI involved, review and approval procedures utilized (i.e., full or expedited review under either federal human research policies or Privacy Rule regulations) and signature by the Chair or other designated member of the reviewing board.

Waivers are likely to be sought for retrospective studies involving medical records review or database research involving PHI (where the patient is unavailable to give Authorization).

An IRB or Privacy Board may also grant a "partial waiver," as defined in Department of Health and Human Services (DHHS) commentary. The partial waiver can be granted separately—even if the IRB/Privacy Board does not grant a waiver of informed consent to participate in the research or a Waiver for access to PHI. Partial waivers are likely to be sought to enable investigators to contact and recruit individuals as potential research subjects. The PHI to be shared would be limited to that necessary to determine eligibility.

Impact on Patient Recruitment

Recruiting subjects includes both the challenge of getting the information to the potential recruits and getting them interested in the study. It is important to remember that a research Authorization under the HIPAA Privacy Rule only permits the use and disclosure of PHI created for research. If a covered entity has an existing relationship with the patient and wants to use or disclose the PHI it obtained prior to the research for determining eligibility, separate Authorization (or Waiver) may be required. Methods for the identification of potential subjects and recruitment must be included in the IRB application to review the research.

Investigators typically find their research patients in one of three ways:
1. Identifying patients from within their own patient database,
2. Seeking and obtaining referrals from other patient databases, or
3. Through advertising and promotion (newspapers, radio, TV, etc.).

The current number of subjects participating in trials within a given disease category remains incredibly low, and many current recruitment strategies are focused on reaching individuals who have never considered clinical research as a healthcare option.

The key consideration in determining how to use PHI appropriately is whether the basic overriding purpose of the Privacy Rule is upheld. The overriding intent of the Privacy Rule is to give individuals power over the discretionary use and dispersal of their health information. An approach may not technically violate the Privacy Rule but if it results in use/disclosure of PHI beyond patients' express permission and where no other exceptions apply, it is not appropriate. The discussion that follows presents examples of acceptable management of PHI for current recruitment and retention strategies under the Privacy Rule.

Identifying Patients for a Study Within the Investigator's Practice (within the covered entity)

The provision for review of PHI preparatory to research allows investigators to access and review their own patients' PHI to determine which patients might be eligible for a trial. Removal of PHI from the investigator's own covered entity is not permitted. Guidance from the Office of Civil Rights (OCR), assigned the task of enforcing compliance with the Privacy Rule, confirms that a researcher or other member of the covered entity's workforce may use PHI to contact prospective subjects. Because HIPAA does not limit disclosures to patients about their own information, covered entities may continue to discuss the option of enrolling in a clinical trial without an

Authorization or Waiver. However, the covered entity's Privacy Notice must mention its intent to use/disclose PHI for this purpose.

Identifying individuals who may be appropriate for selected trials is sometimes delegated to other parties in order to reduce investigators' administrative burden of identifying records that pass the initial screening. This task can be delegated to an outside organization—even to study sponsors—by providing "de-identified" patient data. To be "de-identified," health information must not include any of 18 types of identifiers (e.g., name and contact information, dates [except year], Social Security number, medical record or plan beneficiary number, URLs, email or IP addresses). The sponsor does not receive any information or combination of information that could reveal the patient's identity. Each patient record contains a code that would allow only the investigator to re-identify the patient PHI. After screening the data, the sponsor provides the investigator with a report confirming those records that passed the initial screening. The investigator then re-identifies the subset of patient records, makes an assessment about whether the individuals selected are appropriate candidates and subsequently contacts the patients to find out if they are interested in taking part in the trial.

Delegation strategies encourage those doctors who would otherwise shun the additional administrative work of clinical trials to participate as investigators. While the local patient base within each investigator's organization remains limited, this strategy increases the patient bases by increasing the number of investigators.

Referrals from Other Physicians

It is common for investigators to ask their colleagues for assistance in identifying patients eligible for clinical trials. The most common approach targets specific patients: a treating physician reviews patient charts or a clinical data repository from his/her own covered entity against the study entry criteria and identifies patients meeting the criteria. If this PHI is shared between covered entities, it is a disclosure that triggers Privacy Rule protections. The investigator must determine that the referring physician has obtained either Authorizations from referred patients or a Waiver for this specific purpose.

It is the treating physician's responsibility to obtain patient Authorizations or a Waiver from his/her own IRB/Privacy Board to share PHI outside his/her covered entity. The Authorization may also include permission for the investigator to contact the patient. The treating physician should usually make the initial contact. Patients expect that information on their medical condition will be kept confidential. Many would consider it a serious breach of confidentiality to be contacted by someone not involved in his/her care.

Interestingly, the Privacy Rule allows for a Waiver to share PHI to be granted by the requesting investigator's IRB/Privacy Board. Yet this is a bit like "the fox watching the hen house." The treating physician's covered entity is not bound to accept it and may make its own evaluation.

Referral Letters

To facilitate referrals, an investigator may ask treating physicians to send out letters to their patients describing the study. The investigator's IRB must approve any such patient letter prior to use.

Many referral letters introduce the study to eligible patients and invite them to contact someone in the treating physician's office (which has an existing relationship with the patient) who can provide them with more information about the study. If the patient is interested in being referred to the study, his/her Authorization is required for the treating physician to share the patient's PHI with the investigator.

If the treating physician directs the letter to patients identified through record review, the treating physician's Privacy Notice must mention its intent to use/disclose PHI for this purpose. However, if the treating physician's office sends the letter to all patients—not just those identified by record review—and the investigator has no access to the list of recipients, no Privacy Rule protections are triggered. The letter may provide the investigator's contact information to allow patient self-referral and is thus analogous to any other "non-targeted" advertisement.

"Honest Brokers"

An "honest broker" may serve as an intermediary to facilitate patient referral. To identify eligible patients, an honest broker can de-identify PHI and code it in such a way that it can be re-identified. The investigator reviews the de-identified information to determine which patients meet study criteria. Since de-identified data are exempt, this part of the procedure would not require prior Authorization by patients. The broker then re-identifies the patients meeting the study criteria and provides the names of the identified patients to their personal physician(s). The patients' personal physician contacts the patients to introduce the study, ascertains their interest and obtains Authorization to share their PHI and be contacted by the investigator(s). The honest broker must be an agent of the referring covered entity and he or she cannot be one of the research investigators.

Data Mining

Data mining involves the analysis of claims and or clinical data using algorithms to identity and target potential participants with conditions of interest. It is broadly used for outcomes research but is increasingly being applied to recruitment for clinical trials. For example, a diabetes disease claims search would target patients who have prescriptions for insulin or blood sugar pills or have been admitted to the hospital with a diabetic crisis. Data mining can be executed on local or national databases, such as from a pharmacy benefits management company, the collection of several clinic, pharmacy and hospital databases that exist under the umbrella of a health system or an independent commercial organization (data mining company). Data mining for identification of potential clinical trial participants can generate a list of potential participants who meet a study's age and gender requirements, have already been screened for inclusions and exclusions and are in the same geographic area as various study sites. The doctors conducting the study could then be provided with a list of their own patients who fit the study protocol.

Disclosure of PHI by a non-covered entity is not subject to the Privacy Rule, so an investigator receiving such a list (PHI) could contact individuals to discuss the research study provided that this use has been disclosed in his/her entity's Privacy Notice. Under the Privacy Rule PHI may be used within a covered entity, so the same is true when such a list is generated and provided to an investigator within the same covered entity. However, if the organization mining the data is a covered entity separate from the investigators', providing the list for the purpose of research recruitment is a Privacy Rule disclosure that requires prior Authorization or a Waiver, even if the data are about the investigators' own patients.

Advertising and Promotion

Recruitment advertisements appear in newspapers, on public transportation, on radio and television as well as on the Internet. The recruitment advertising may be managed by individual investigators or by central "recruitment centers." Recruitment centers publish advertising/websites that focus on symptoms and treatment for certain diseases/conditions. They distribute information to patients, caregivers and advocacy groups about clinical trials that are currently recruiting patients. Patients may "opt-in" and register (voluntarily providing identifiable health information) with these centers to receive information on clinical trials (and may "opt-out" at any time). Registered patients respond to the center if they are interested in a specific trial and may be referred directly to an investigator or to someone at the recruitment center who may administer a trial-specific screening interview. Alternatively, the center may transmit identifiable health information to investigators allowing them to make subsequent patient contact. This disclosure is not appropriate unless the recruitment company has obtained the patients' prior permission to transmit this information to a clinical site. Covered entities must obtain this permission in the form of a written Authorization. However for non-covered entities, obtaining verbal permission is currently sufficient.

Even though the Privacy Rule may not apply (many recruitment centers are non-covered entities), federal human research policies remain in effect. For instance, federal human research policies consider advertisements and screening interviews/scripts to be part of the informed consent process, which therefore must be approved by the governing IRB(s) prior to use.

Potential Patient Initiates Contact

Most advertising campaigns result in the interested, potential recruit contacting the investigator. These respondents have initiated the first contact and have, therefore, implicitly given their permission to be contacted by study staff. Because HIPAA does not limit disclosures to individuals of their own information, once contact is made, the investigator or study staff may discuss the option of enrolling in the clinical trial without an Authorization or Waiver.

However, if the next step for the investigator is to conduct a screening interview that results in PHI from potential patients being recorded prior to administration of the research Authorization/consent, then the investigator must obtain an Authorization or be granted a partial waiver for this use. If an IRB is presented a screening script for review, it makes sense for the IRB to evaluate its acceptability in terms of the criteria required to grant a Waiver. The IRB can grant a "partial waiver" for use of the PHI collected at the same time it grants IRB approval for the actual script.

Investigator Initiates Contact

A recruitment center may pass a pre-screened list of candidates' (PHI) on to the investigator for the investigator to initiate contact. If a recruitment center is a covered entity, Authorization is required for the PHI to pass to the investigator. However, Privacy Rule protections are triggered only if the recruitment center is a covered entity—and many are not.

If the recruitment center is a covered entity, then the investigator must ensure that a) the recruitment center has obtained appropriate Authorizations under the Privacy Rule, or b) the recruitment center's IRB or Privacy Board has issued a Waiver for this specific disclosure and contact.

If the recruitment center is not a covered entity, then the Privacy Rule does not apply. The PHI may pass to the investigator without Authorization or Waiver; and the investigator may contact the recruits, who have initiated the first contact and voluntarily contributed information. This is a form of self-referral. In this context, the provisions of the Privacy Rule do not apply until the investigator intends to record PHI for the research.

Special Events

Recruitment strategies often include disseminating information through speaking engagements with professional or community organizations, patient associations and advocacy groups, or health fairs and medical screenings.

Investigators or recruitment centers draw an audience at health fairs by offering blood pressure checks, asthma screening, computer-assisted cancer, stroke and heart disease risk assessments, cholesterol blood tests, as well as pediatric height and weight checks, etc. Educational material and clinical trial advertising are distributed. Covered entities must make a Privacy Notice available and obtain acknowledgement in order to record test results or contact patients regarding results that cannot be provided immediately.

Patients may refer themselves to clinical studies in response to these efforts. By contrast, recording PHI in order to contact patients regarding research studies is considered building a research database and covered entities must obtain patient Authorization for this purpose.

Use and Maintenance of Recruitment Databases

Whether by an individual investigator or recruitment center, the creation of a clinical trial database containing a few, but vital, pieces of information, including different chronic ailments, is a very useful tool maintained by continuously adding new information.

Referred potential patients do not always meet study entry criteria or are not interested in a particular study. De-identified information regarding non-enrollers, including the number of inquiries, screening appointments and disqualifications is not subject to the Privacy Rule and can be kept along with the reasons for disqualifications or refusal. Yet recruiters may also want to keep the PHI from non-enrollers in order to contact patients about participation in future studies. Covered entities must obtain written Authorization or a Waiver to do so. Oral Authorization is not valid for them; therefore it cannot be obtained by telephone as part of a screening interview. Recruitment centers are typically non-covered entities and can, however, obtain this permission verbally by telephone or through the Internet. Recruitment activities of non-covered entities are not affected unless they involve access to PHI controlled by a covered entity. Consequently, these centers are able to offer investigators access to much larger and more comprehensive databases containing patient information.

Patient Retention

While the focus thus far has been on patient recruitment, patient retention in a clinical trial can ultimately be more important, particularly in long-term trials. A high dropout rate can add delay or cause a study to fail completely. Retention and compliance are supported by appointment reminders, compliance monitoring and drug reminder calls. Patients in clinical trials remain motivated through one-on-one contact and communication about what they can expect and their responsibilities in the study and through continued positive reinforcement. Happily, this is consistent with the concept of informed consent as an ongoing process. Yet, the skilled and consistent execution of these tasks over time is a serious resource concern for investigative sites.

The use of centralized retention services, contributing efficiency and core competence is also the current trend in this area. Investigators must disclose PHI to organizations providing patient retention services to allow their interaction with study participants during a clinical trial. This disclosure can be made as long as it is anticipated and represented in the patient's Authorization to use and disclose PHI for the clinical trial.

Summary

Eighty percent of clinical trials suffer delay or failure because of inadequate patient recruitment. To overcome this statistic, both government and private industry are taking action to increase public awareness and trust of clinical trials. Patient retention is equally or more important than patient recruitment for the success of clinical trials. The responsibility for patient recruitment and retention is shifting from the individual investigators to centralized recruitment campaigns and retention services. These efforts must comply with the Privacy Rule regarding the use and disclosure of PHI.

The Privacy Rule is supplemental to existing regulations and impacts the actions of covered entities, and sometimes affects the interactions between covered entities and recruitment centers, regarding exchange of PHI.

Key Takeaways

- The HIPAA Privacy Rule applies to the clinical trial recruitment activities of covered entities, i.e., most investigators.
- The HIPAA Privacy Rule does not apply to non-covered entities, i.e., most recruitment organizations. Recruitment activities of non-covered entities are not affected unless they involve access to PHI controlled by a covered entity.
- The overriding intent of the Privacy Rule is to give individuals power over the discretionary use and dispersal of their health information.
- You can check whether your recruitment strategy is appropriate under the Privacy Rule by determining whether the basic overriding purpose of the Privacy Rule is upheld.

- Where the Privacy Rule and federal human research policies (45 CFR 46, 21 CFR 50 and 56) are applicable, both must be followed. Where they overlap, the most stringent standard applies. Some states also have laws that address disclosure of information that may be more stringent than the Privacy Rule. If this is the case, then state law will prevail.

References

Code of Federal Regulations, Title 45, Part 160 and 164 (U.S. Government Printing Office, Washington, DC).

Code of Federal Regulations, Title 45, Part 46 (U.S. Government Printing Office, Washington, DC).

Code of Federal Regulations, Title 21, Part 50 (U.S. Government Printing Office, Washington, DC).

Code of Federal Regulations, Title 21, Part 56 (U.S. Government Printing Office, Washington, DC).

Office of Civil Rights, OCR Guidance Explaining Significant Aspects of the Privacy Rule (OCR, Washington, DC, December 2002). Also available at www.hhs.gov/ocr/hipaa/privacy.html.

Author Biographies

Ellen Kelso Holt
Founder, Goodwyn Institutional Review Board, Ltd.
Ellen Kelso Holt has over 23 years of experience in clinical research and regulatory affairs. Ms. Holt founded Goodwyn Institutional Review Board, Ltd. (Goodwyn IRB) in 1999. She is a certified IRB professional and for the past five years has served as Goodwyn IRB's Administrative Vice-Chair and Managing Member.

Prior to her work with Goodwyn IRB, Ms. Holt served Kendle International (a Cincinnati-based clinical research organization) as Assistant Director of Regulatory Affairs responsible for clinical research site selection, coordination of documents for initiation and execution of large-scale clinical trials, and clinical trial quality control.

Before Kendle, she spent three years at Procter & Gamble Pharmaceuticals as Regulatory Affairs and Standards Manager. While at P&GP she led project teams through production and approval of new drug applications (NDAs), managed international submission strategies and established electronic submission publication, document management and regulatory compliance systems.

Ms. Holt began her career at Eli Lilly and Company planning and spent over thirteen years administering clinical trials, preparing international regulatory submissions and safety reporting. She was also the company's world-wide regulatory point-person for human insulin products. She has authored (or co-authored) articles and book chapters focusing on various topics in drug development safety reporting and human subject protections in research. She has been a consultant in the design and support for research program training for investigators, study coordinators, IRB staff and members.

Sheila Elliott Kinney, J.D.

Sheila Elliott Kinney earned her law degree from Indiana University and has practiced both with a private law firm and in the public sector representing various governmental agencies. She has significant experience advising clients on a broad array of operational issues including HIPAA assessment. Ms. Kinney serves as a member of the Goodwyn Institutional Review Board.

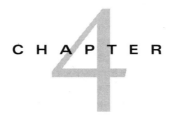

CHAPTER 4

Facilitating Best Practices: The Need for Standard Operating Procedures and Ongoing Training

Diana L. Anderson, Ph.D., D. Anderson & Company
Nanette Myers, B.S., D. Anderson & Company

Objectives
- Define best practices as related to patient recruitment.
- Identify standard operating procedures (SOPs) and training as key elements of best practices for research organizations.
- Present various types of recruitment SOPs and explain the implementation process.
- Explain the critical importance of training investigative sites to think beyond the in-house patient database as a referral source by considering a wide array of recruitment techniques to attract targeted populations.
- Discuss the trend toward involving sponsors in the training process as they recognize the value of having sites trained in patient recruitment.

Introduction

The development and implementation of best practices have long been recognized in the corporate world as key to an organization's ongoing success. In the young clinical trials market, best practices is a fairly new concept, and within the patient recruitment niche, the idea is just starting to take root.

Best practices are proven methods and processes employed by companies to maximize strategic, operational and financial advantage.[1] They are important drivers of success because they enable a company or department to achieve best results by using standardized, consistent and effective methodologies.[2]

The best practices approach holds promise for the improvement of patient recruitment activities undertaken by research organizations such as sponsors, contract research organizations (CROs), site management organizations (SMOs), and particularly the investigative site where many of the recruitment activities take place. With the help of best practices, the site can move away from haphazard recruitment efforts that are reinvented with each study and start moving toward a systematic approach that has focus, goals and an infrastructure that acknowledges the complexities of patient recruitment and its relationship to patient retention.

Best practices in patient recruitment involves taking a comprehensive approach that includes many factors such as identifying recruitment and retention obstacles, identifying motivators and public perceptions that have an impact on clinical trial participation, and developing effective advertising messages and materials. By adopting these techniques, it is possible to lay the foundation for benchmarking, which is the process of identifying, using, and sharing best practices to improve business processes within the organization.[3]

Benchmarking can make a powerful impact on an organization because it creates a learning culture, enables readiness for action and provides models of excellence that allow a company to continuously improve. Companies benchmark in an attempt to accelerate and manage change, to make better-informed decisions, incorporate innovations, create a sense of urgency, overcome complacency, understand world-class performance and improve profits.[4]

The elements of best practices and benchmarking are articulated in the form of standard operating procedures (SOPs). Without written SOPs, best practices remain mostly theoretical and are difficult to implement because they are subject to individual interpretations. Well-written SOPs offer users a clear directive for translating best practices into action.

This chapter is dedicated to highlighting how and why SOPs facilitate best practices that make a difference in patient recruitment activities across the clinical research enterprise. Equally important is identifying the need for ongoing training in patient recruitment techniques as a best practice. As the demand for study volunteers increases, sites will be less likely to meet their recruitment goals from internal databases and non-focused advertising. Site staff need training in the use of more sophisticated tools and planning techniques that can assist in the meeting of enrollment targets and the boosting of retention rates.

Developing Standard Operating Procedures (SOPs)

Best practices in patient recruitment start with standardizing recruitment processes that can be measured against proven strategies. This metrics-based scientific approach is facilitated by the development and implementation of

SOPs. As recruitment challenges grow along with the number of clinical trials and the number of patients needed per trial (Table 1), introducing standardized practices is the first step toward measuring outcomes and overcoming recruitment obstacles resulting from inexperience, lack of organization and reactive planning.

Table 1: Recruitment Challenges

- 80,000—estimated number of ongoing trials
- 5,300—average number of patients per new drug application (NDA)
- 14%—percentage of studies in which enrollment is completed on schedule
- 81%—percentage of studies in which enrollment is delayed one to six months
- 85%—percentage of Americans diagnosed with a life-threatening illness, such as cancer, who reported that they were either unaware of clinical trials or weren't sure that they were an option

Source: CenterWatch, Harris Interactive Surveys

SOPs identify the various recruitment-related tasks and specify how they are to be done and who has the responsibility. Because adherence to well thought out SOPs is pivotal to a successful organization, training on SOPs should be an integral part of new employee training, and part of ongoing training for existing employees. Creation and implementation of SOPs, coupled with proper training, will allow for a better understanding of the roles of each member of the research team and encourage improved compliance with the U.S. Food and Drug Administration (FDA), Department of Health and Human Services (HHS), and International Conference on Harmonisation (ICH) guidelines. Planning and training of this type are no longer casual options. They are good business practices and are critical to recruitment success.

Developing the SOP is best accomplished by using a template that lists its various elements. The elements, or sections, of the SOP include its **purpose, policy, references** and **appendices** (as in Table 2). Using the direct mail SOP as an example, the purpose may read, "To describe the procedures followed by ABC Company when implementing a direct mail campaign to recruit study participants."

Next is the policy section. It is generally the lengthiest as it contains the meat of the SOP, defining exactly how a task is to be completed. It also includes any associated definitions. The direct mail SOP, for example, explains that this modality is often used in recruitment campaigns and that direct mail comprises internal and external mailing categories. It then defines internal and external mail and describes aspects relating to external

---

Table 2: ABC Company, SOP No. 008—Direct Mail Campaign

I. Purpose

To describe the procedures followed by ABC Company when implementing a direct mail campaign to recruit study participants

II. Policy

Direct Mail Campaign: Direct mail campaigns are often included in the ABC proposals to identify potential study participants. ABC creates, produces and distributes the direct mail pieces. Below are the details outlining each of these steps along with the different types of direct mail campaigns.

    A. **Internal Mailing:** There are two different types of direct mail that may be used, internal and external. The internal direct mail utilizes the data that ABC has built by entering patients that consent to being contacted for future trials, by using an opt in process, of which they might qualify. The consent/opt in process that we use is HIPAA-compliant because the individuals themselves are voluntarily requesting contact for future trials

    B. **External Mailing:** ABC works with numerous different mailing list providers to conduct an external direct mail campaign. These companies identify patients that may qualify for study participation by analyzing the inclusion and exclusion criteria for the corresponding therapeutic indication and the location of these individuals to the research sites

        1) **Creation:** The information that is included on the direct mail piece corresponds with the other recruitment materials, graphically

Source: D. Anderson & Co.

direct mail, such as creation and production of the mail piece. It also mentions that external mailings include the purchase of lists of potential study subjects.

The policy section is followed by the reference section, which denotes specific regulatory guidelines, guidances, books that are referenced in the policy section, or other SOPs that relate to the SOP in question. There are three regulatory references for direct mail. They refer to an SOP for the institutional review board (IRB), a reference to FDA Information Sheets, and Section 3.1.2 of the International Conference on Harmonisation guidelines.

The SOP concludes with the appendix section which, in this instance, includes examples of direct mail pieces.

and verbally, that have previously been created for the trial. The text is very similar to the print advertising text, but also includes a perforated reply card. This reply card allows the potential study subjects to mail their information to ABC consenting to be contacted for study screening. After creation and sponsor approval, the direct mail piece is then forwarded to the IRB for approval prior to production.

2) **Production:** ABC may utilize the services of one of many of its outside vendors for printing of the direct mail piece. The amount to be printed is identified in the proposal process.

3) **List Purchase and Distribution:** When conducting an external mailing, ABC will purchase list(s) from an outside vendor. These clearinghouse companies have identified potential study participants through market research surveys. Based on the study criteria, including disease indication, age, and the geographic location to the research center, a list is generated with the appropriate number of individuals to which the direct mail piece will be mailed. The list company then mails this piece to the corresponding individuals.

III. References
See IRB SOP
FDA Information Sheets
ICH Section 3.1.2

IV. Appendices
Direct Mail Example Attached

It is good form to create a title page for each SOP containing the name and number of the SOP. The title page should be signed and dated by one or more company officials. A signed, dated title page is a handy way to let the reader know that he or she is reading the latest version of the SOP. So, if an organization reviews and updates SOPs annually, the dates and signatures on the cover page should be fairly recent. For reference purposes, companies may choose to keep older versions of SOPs or deleted ones, but they should be marked as "historic" or "void" to clearly show that they are no longer in effect.

Once SOPs have been written for each process that the research organization believes should be documented, a table of contents is created. It should list the title of each SOP, in order of appearance.

Finally, the SOP documents are either printed and placed in a binder that is easily accessible, or uploaded to a secured intranet Web site. For organizations that maintain intranet Web sites, it is a good idea to keep a printed SOP binder for quick access, as there may be times when a desktop computer or a wireless personal digital assistant is inaccessible or inconvenient.

Company SOPs are often confidential documents; therefore, groups using printed binders may want to implement sign in and sign out sheets to document who has the binder(s). When SOPs are available on a company intranet, the user would gain access and be identified by password.

Implementation

Standard operating procedures are living processes that attest to an organization's commitment to best practices and benchmarking. Generally, they are developed by teams with a stake in seeing the SOPs serve as a foundation for success. For this reason, it is critical that the research staff be made aware of the SOPs and be included in the implementation process.

To implement newly written or revised SOPs, staff members should receive advance notice and adequate time to read them. Next, management should schedule one or more training sessions, depending on the size of the organization. Throughout the training process, staff must receive consistent messages that SOPs are guidelines with a purpose, and that they are not just suggestions, and, therefore, must be followed.

To encourage buy-in, it is important to ask for questions and solicit honest feedback. Acknowledge that a special circumstance or request for an exception to the SOP can be presented through the exception request process, which must be approved.

To keep the SOPs current, one or more staff members should be designated to maintain and update the SOPs as part of their job responsibilities. For most organizations, SOPs should be reviewed by the designated parties on an annual basis for relevance, accuracy and comprehension. As part of this process, organizations may want to encourage staff input as to whether one or more of the SOPs are outdated or impractical.

Once an SOP is edited, a new title page that is signed and dated by the appropriate officer should be placed on the SOP to indicate it is the most recent version of the policy. In addition, copies of the revised SOP might be circulated to the staff for their review and, depending on the extent of change, one-on-one or group training and discussion should occur.

Various Types of SOPs

If SOPs are the vehicles through which best practices are expressed, it is important to identify those processes requiring SOPs. Within the realm of clinical practice, there are a whole host of processes to document, ranging from administrative tasks, regulatory affairs, study startup and data management to quality assurance, etc.[5] In the patient recruitment niche, there are a number of SOPs that highlight the growing number of tools needed to launch an effective campaign. These include FDA regulatory compliance of recruitment materials, recruitment web site SOP, HIPAA SOP and more (see Table 3).

Table 3: Some Recruitment SOPs

- FDA regulatory compliance of recruitment materials
- Recruitment web site
- Call center/prescreening
- Metrics collection
- Health Insurance Portability and Accountability Act (HIPAA)
- Direct mail
- Creation and production of recruitment materials

Source: D. Anderson & Co.

FDA Regulatory Compliance of Recruitment Materials SOP

Abiding by the FDA regulations as spelled out in various sections of Title 21 Code of Federal Regulations (CFR) is mandatory for conducting quality research in accordance with Good Clinical Practice (GCP). The details of operating in GCP mode are to be described in an organization's SOPs.

CFR regulations do not actually state that recruitment materials must be reviewed by an accredited IRB; however, this is standard practice among sponsors and well-run investigative sites and is the result of statements from FDA Information Sheets that provide guidance to IRBs and clinical investigators. In an Information Sheet entitled "Recruiting Study Subjects,"[6] there are various statements describing the IRB's responsibilities to review the methods and materials that investigators propose to use to recruit subjects. This includes direct advertising that is intended to be seen or heard by prospective subjects to solicit their participation in a study, and refers to, but is not limited to, newspaper advertising; radio and TV scripts, along with audio and video (TV); Internet postings, bulletin boards, posters, doctor-to-patient letters, and flyers that are intended for prospective subjects.

Additionally, according to this FDA Information Sheet, the agency considers the direct advertising for study subjects to be the start of the informed consent and subject selection process. In following this line of thinking, FDA guidelines definitely come into play. CFR Part 50 Subpart B addresses elements of informed consent, and appropriate parts of this reference should be stated in the reference portion of the SOP.

The International Conference on Harmonisation does specifically comment on the review of recruitment materials by an accredited ethics review committee in Section 3.1.2, which describes responsibilities of IRBs and independent ethics committees (IECs). The section mentions that IRBs and IECs are to obtain recruitment materials, as described in Table 4.

Table 4: ICH Good Clinical Practice Guideline 3.1.2

"The IRB/IEC should obtain the following documents:

Trial protocol(s)/amendments, written informed consent form(s) and consent form updates that the investigator proposes for use in the trial, subject recruitment procedures (e.g., advertisements), written information to be provided to subjects, Investigator's Brochure (IB), available safety information...."

FDA guidelines address the issue of document storage for a specified length of time. All of the IRB-approved recruitment materials, including signed and dated informed consent documents, should be stored in the regulatory binder and kept for the required length of time as stated in CFR Part 312.62(c). This guideline mentions that the record retention period is two years following the date of approval of a marketing application; or if no application is made, or if the application is not approved, until two years after the investigation is discontinued and FDA is notified.

The SOP outlining the review of recruitment materials should include:

- The IRB submission process for all recruitment materials.
- Storage and maintenance guidelines for these documents.

Recruitment Web Site SOP

Recruitment web sites are growing in popularity as a recruitment device. CenterWatch market research indicates that 85% of the top 25 pharma/biotech companies were recruiting patients online in 2003, and more than 12,000 trials were listed through www.centerwatch.com, up 25%

from 2002.[7] Approximately 30,000 site trials were listed with the National Institutes of Health (NIH) or the National Cancer Institute (NCI). This heavy reliance on the Internet mirrors the boom in web browsing for health information, an activity engaged in by some 73 million Americans, according to the 2002 Pew Internet and American Life Project.[8]

Recruitment web sites run the gamut from simple to more complex. Some function as trial listing services with contact information while others allow potential participants to pre-screen for study participation. Consequently, the SOP for a recruitment web site will vary depending on the web site's degree of sophistication and on whether a potential subject's health information is passed from a "non-covered entity" to a "covered entity" under the HIPAA Privacy Rule.

The SOP may discuss:

- A description of the web site and its uses. A study-specific web site, for example, will educate the public on the disease indication, describe applicable clinical trials, and may allow viewers to pre-screen qualify. A web site for a clinical trial site may have a brief description of the trials in progress and those that are still recruiting, and may list a few key inclusion/exclusion criteria along with a contact telephone number.
- How individuals handling the recruitment web site should identify industry web sites to which it should be hyperlinked. The SOP should also discuss how to gain permission to include those industry web links on the recruitment web site.
- The security measures that are in place to maintain the confidentiality of any information entered onto the web site.
- The sponsor approval process of the web site followed by submission to an accredited IRB.
- The measures that are in place to comply with the HIPAA Privacy Rule, if a potential subject's personal health information will be transferred from a "non-covered entity" to a "covered entity." (See "HIPAA Privacy Rule SOP Specific to Patient Recruitment" in this chapter.)

This SOP should reflect the level of detail and sophistication of the web site. There will be substantial differences between an SOP for a detailed, study-specific web site and one containing simple trial listings on an organization's web site.

Pre-Screening/Call Center SOP

This SOP outlines how the pre-screening process should be conducted and includes details of operating the call center for those research organizations with call center capability. Recent data suggest an increase in spending on call centers, particularly central ones, with annual growth projected in the low double digits. Research indicates that spending on central call centers reached an estimated $120 million in 2003.[9] With these large sums at stake, it is important to detail the best practices for the answering of telephones, pre-screening of potential subjects and a metric for responding to emails and voice mail messages so that all calls are returned promptly and courteously within a certain time frame.

The pre-screening/call center SOP may include:

- The development and approval process of the pre-screening questionnaire
- The designation of one or more phone lines, whether a toll-free or local number, for recruitment
- The hours when staff or operators are available to answer the dedicated recruitment line(s)
- The process by which the information is collected (electronic/hard copy) and how it is stored including the security measures surrounding this confidential information
- The process by which a potential subject's personal health information is transferred from a "non-covered entity" to a "covered entity" in accordance with the HIPAA Privacy Rule, if applicable.
- A metric for responding to email and voice mail messages. Suggested time frames are 24 to 48 hours for an email response, and 24 hours for a voicemail response.

Metrics Collection SOP

The collection of metrics, which begins with the first phone call or Internet screen, entails measuring and analyzing the success of various patient recruitment initiatives. Metrics collection is critical because it enables the staff to identify what's working and what isn't and allows for a quick refocusing of methods to maximize recruitment dollars.

Determining the best way to collect metrics adds a scientific element to the recruitment process because it enables the research organization to make decisions about the success of patient recruitment activities based on proven methodology and hard data, instead of speculation. Collecting metrics leads to the building of databases with historical information, which allows for analysis of what works in various geographic areas for specific disease indications.

This SOP addresses how to collect metrics and how to utilize the resulting data to make decisions about an ongoing recruitment campaign.

Guidelines that may be included in the metric collection SOP are:

- Determining the source of the screening information, for instance, the telephone and Internet pre-screening questionnaires might start by asking the potential candidate how he or she learned about the study

- Detailing what is done with the information once it is collected
- Describing how the data will be used to drive the current and future patient recruitment campaigns

HIPAA Privacy Rule SOP Specific to Patient Recruitment

Compliance with HIPAA, or the Health Insurance Portability and Accountability Act of 1996, is a complex subject that is covered in detail in Chapter 3, but for the purposes of an SOP discussion, it is worth commenting on HIPAA's impact on patient recruitment and how that impact is reflected in an organization's SOPs.

Clinical research falls under the Privacy Rule regulation of HIPAA, which establishes minimum federal standards for the protection of certain personal health information of living or deceased individuals. Clinical investigators may be affected directly or indirectly by the Privacy Rule if their research requires the use of, or access to, an individual's identifiable health information, known as protected health information, or PHI. Investigators should be aware of the Privacy Rule because it establishes the conditions under which *covered entities* can have access to or disclose PHI for many purposes, such as clinical research.[10] This includes activities such as subject screening and recruitment.[11]

A *covered entity* is either a healthcare provider who transmits information electronically in connection with transactions for which the Department of Health and Human Services (HHS) has adopted standards, a health plan payor, or a healthcare clearinghouse. Investigators may be or may work for a covered entity; therefore, they need to understand the Privacy Rule which describes how covered entities can establish relationships in which PHI can be used and shared, and under what conditions it can allow use of or disclosure of the information.

When drafting an SOP to describe the proper handling of PHI, a research organization must first determine whether it is a covered entity. It is recommended that a group consult an attorney to learn if it is a covered entity and to understand how or if it is to comply with the Privacy Rule. Information about the Privacy Rule is available at http://privacyrule andresearch.nih.gov/pr_02.asp.

Non-covered entities, such as some CROs, recruitment providers and site management organizations (SMOs), may have access to identifiable health information and therefore may want to adopt SOPs that are similar to those implemented by covered entities. For example, a non-covered entity, such as a recruitment provider, may choose not to accept lists of potential study candidates that come from the databases of investigative sites. Non-covered entities may choose not to do any mailings to individuals who pre-screen on a Web site.

Below are general guidelines.

- The SOP should state if the organization is a covered entity.
- The SOP should describe how the organization gains access to PHI, i.e., does the PHI come from recruitment advertising?
- Potential study volunteers responding to advertising should grant approval to the research entity to enter PHI into a patient database.
- Once the PHI is collected, how is it handled, and to whom is it sent, i.e., sponsor, CRO?
- Describe the security measures that individuals must follow to gain access to the PHI, such as log-in passwords that are changed periodically.
- Describe how PHI is secured, including physical security for paper copies, electronic security for Web-based information, and data backup.
- What security features does the patient database include, especially if it is accessed via the Internet? This discussion addresses logon identifier-expiration time frames, and inactive termination settings to prevent PHI from long-term visibility on a computer screen.

The Need for Staff Training in Patient Recruitment

Operating in best practices mode is about more than drafting and implementing well thought out SOPs. There are many elements to the clinical trials process, ranging from the informed consent process to final billing, and all are ripe for the establishment of best practices and benchmarks. Included in this list should be ongoing staff training in how to conduct effective patient recruitment and retention campaigns.

The traditional patient recruitment model has centered on sponsors' continual reliance on investigators who have proven that they can recruit a negotiated number of study subjects from within their own practices and networks. Historically, this method was successful as studies were somewhat limited in size, and scope, and to a handful of key investigators. But, since the early 1990s, the clinical trials industry has transitioned into a bigger, more complex multi-site global enterprise, demanding ever more volunteers, and decreasing the likelihood that investigators will be able to continue enrolling the contracted number of patients from their private practices.

As the search for study candidates intensifies, investigators and sponsors are recognizing that they need to hone new skill sets and competencies to achieve enrollment targets. This means moving beyond the tried and true processes of manual chart review and scouring the internal database in favor of a broader range of resources, namely multi-media advertising, central call centers, central ad campaigns, Internet postings, direct mail and more. Evidence suggests that this movement is well under way as various types of investigative sites are relying more frequently on promotional efforts (see Table 5).[12] What is not clear is to what extent these efforts are successful.

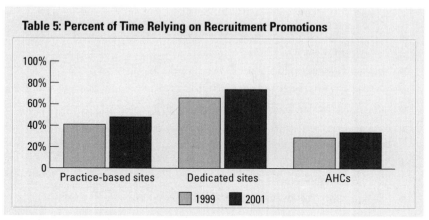

Table 5: Percent of Time Relying on Recruitment Promotions

Source: CenterWatch, 2003

According to federal regulations, sponsors are to select only those investigators who are qualified by training and experience to study a compound.[13] The challenge is that generally, those same clinical experts have limited, if any, experience in mounting comprehensive recruitment campaigns to supplement enrollment. Training in this critical aspect of clinical development, whether in a classroom setting, self-paced online mode, a live online session, or at regional or national industry meetings, becomes a key best practice supporting the mission of bringing innovative therapies to market sooner.

Training in best recruitment practices is built on some basic common sense principles such as ensuring the staff understands the protocol and procedures; achieving consensus and agreement on recruitment initiatives; obtaining commitment on scheduling and follow-up; and encouraging site staff to read literature about the condition being studied. With these building blocks in place, patient recruitment training teaches a wide range of strategies that address project feasibility, resource planning, return-on-investment (ROI) assessment, regulations, ethical issues and media planning (see Table 6).

Training should also explore the benefits of centralized recruitment initiatives, help sites build successful strategies of their own, address the critical link between good customer service and retention, and review the informed consent process as the start of the recruitment effort. The goal of the training is to orient the staff toward taking a proactive stance, instead of defaulting to seat-of-the-pants advertising tactics in a desperate attempt to boost enrollment.

Table 6: Some Best Recruitment Practices©

- Identify recruitment and retention obstacles
- Identify motivators and public perceptions impacting clinical trial participation
- Design effective means to assess site resources and realistically determine enrollment projections
- Develop proactive, customized recruitment and retention plans
- Prioritize recruitment strategies
- Develop effective advertising messages and materials
- Identify challenges when working with third parties and discuss strategies to optimize third party interactions
- Identify ethical, cultural and regulatory considerations that impact recruitment and retention
- Evaluate the effectiveness of recruitment and retention programs

Source: D. Anderson & Co.

Beth Harper, Senior Vice President of Operation at Rheumatology Research International, says that sponsors are becoming more forward thinking about the value of training their investigative sites in patient recruitment methodology, and some are willing to invest the dollars to make this happen. "People are starting to appreciate the complexity of recruitment and the roles they play in the continuum of what recruitment and retention are really all about. Some sponsors are also starting to think beyond the immediate needs of a current study by taking a broader view about how continuous training can help the sites be more successful in the long term," Harper says.

Nothing speaks to a site's commitment to its staff like investing in their training.[14] It shows respect for the professional status of the staff and serves to reduce the overwhelming feelings experienced by study coordinators who may not really understand their responsibilities because they are trained in a rushed, on-the-job manner.

Many sites provide training for study coordinators through certification programs offered by the Association of Clinical Research Professionals (ACRP) and the Society of Clinical Research Association (SOCRA), and while these programs are highly valuable, they focus largely on the principles of Good Clinical Practice, and not necessarily on the specifics of patient recruitment.

Here is where sponsors can step in. According to Harper, "It would serve the industry really well if sponsors could invest in recruitment training, and not just for their immediate studies. Progressive sponsors should be thinking about this investment as a way to get a better pool of qualified sites."

Vicki Johnson, Director of Best Recruitment Practices at D. Anderson & Co., a recruitment provider, says that sponsors often express concern about finding sites able to do a better job of recruiting and retaining subjects. She says, "Ongoing training in this area is definitely indicated and should be considered a best practice. For sponsors willing to make the investment, they are likely to see sites become better trained and more productive in terms of enrollment. They are also likely to see the development of partnerships with those sites."

Partnership building has many benefits for sponsors and sites. Both parties are likely to develop loyalties to each other. Sites may feel a certain allegiance to sponsors who have invested in their training and may favor those sponsors over other sponsors when presented with competitive studies. In becoming a "sponsor of choice," a sponsor may increase its access to well-performing sites that may have benefited from training underwritten by that sponsor.

There are other tangible and intangible benefits linked to recruitment training. Evidence suggests that training improves processes, possibly leads to financial gain; reduces turnover and improves employee morale.[15] According to Johnson, recruitment staff welcomes more education and tools to enhance recruitment initiatives. "The training increases their confidence level and boosts their interest in doing a good job. If the training is supported by a sponsor, they appreciate that the sponsor was interested in making that investment," Johnson explains.

Making Training Effective

Whether training is sponsored by a site or a corporate sponsor, it must be effective and it must be designed to accommodate the needs of sites of various sizes. In today's estimated $4.5 billion study conduct market, part-time investigative sites hold a nearly 40% market share. The other 60% of the market is composed of dedicated sites, academic medical centers and SMOs.[16] These venues have varying degrees of infrastructure, resources, know-how and sophistication.

Larger dedicated sites and SMOs may be positioned to have one or more patient recruiters dedicated to orchestrate and oversee recruitment activities. The other venues generally cannot justify this expense and often add recruitment to the study coordinator's responsibilities.

Toni Brash, President of Brash Consultancy, a training provider, says that sponsors are interested in investing in meaningful training for sites of all sizes. She says, "Sponsors are reaching out to sites of every size and type. Depending on what the site needs, the sponsor may opt to provide workbooks, videos, weekend training in how to recruit, or have a clinical research associate (CRA) trained in patient recruitment dedicate a day onsite. Also, training in the informed consent process remains popular." Brash adds that interactive sessions in which case studies are discussed and sites share tips for success can be effective and more engaging to participants more than a formal lecture format.

Lance Converse, Founder and CEO of ePharmaLearning, a provider of e-learning and e-meeting solutions, agrees that sponsors are interested in training investigative sites of all sizes and are considering both online and face-to-face settings. Converse explains that face-to-face recruitment training works well at investigator meetings at which protocol-specific training takes place. To gain buy-in, he says it is important to encourage a two-way dialogue in which experienced sites have an opportunity to share their knowledge with the sponsor and less experienced sites about which recruitment techniques work and which do not. Converse says, "Sponsors are recognizing that integrating two-way learning with adult learning tools is a best practice. When you enhance buy-in, that's when you get a better response."

At the time of this writing, ePharmaLearning is launching its first e-learning module for patient recruitment. The module is a two-hour program that sites can access on a just-in-time basis, to coincide with the start of a project. With this capability, staff members who are new or have never taken the training course can be trained just as the project begins.

Prior to the product's 2003 launch, Converse conducted an online survey of industry representatives to gauge their level of interest. Of the 300 respondents, most of whom were site selectors, project managers, project directors and investigator recruiters, 94% claimed to believe that an online training module that would teach sites how to be more effective patient recruiters would improve enrollment. Ninety-six percent (96%) responded that they would be willing to underwrite the cost of such training.

As these new training techniques and others come to market, sponsors and sites underwriting the expense will want to know if their investments are effective. They will expect to see metrics supporting a meaningful return-on-investment. Because training in recruitment is quite new and is just taking hold, there are few, if any, metrics, to document success. Toni Brash says, "I don't have any metrics and I haven't been able to find any." Beth Harper agrees with that assessment, "I don't think there are any metrics yet to document success of recruitment training activities. Everyone would like to see an immediate return whereby if they pay to train a site, that will translate into improved patient enrollment right away. I would like to encourage people to take a longer view and look at the benefits of training for the long haul."

The Next Horizon

Using best practices to improve patient recruitment is an approach whose time has come. With recruitment challenges mounting along with the rising number of clinical trials and the demand for study participants, best practices offer tools for turning what can be an overwhelming series of tasks into an organized, professional operation.

Best practices use proven and standardized methods to maximize strategic, operational, and financial advantage, and drive success. In the patient recruitment industry, success is characterized by the consistent meeting of enrollment targets using well-defined, cost-effective and ethical means.

Turning best practices into a practical, hands-on way of doing business is accomplished through the introduction of SOPs that define specifically how the best practices and processes are to be carried out. Without SOPs, it would be difficult to incorporate best practices into the daily routine with any degree of consistency as each staff member would likely have his or her own interpretation.

For research organizations, recruitment SOPs cover the gamut from the creation and production of recruitment materials to details of operating a HIPAA-compliant recruitment web site, to addressing how to collect metrics. To implement the SOPs properly, they need to be presented to the staff in a training session so people are aware of them and can discuss their content. The trainers need to stress that SOPs are guidelines that must be adhered to and are not casual suggestions. Because of their importance, SOPs should be reviewed and updated on a regular, annual basis and should also be part of the training offered to new employees.

Training, itself, is a best practice. Because patient recruitment is a complex enterprise, ongoing training in this critical function is highly indicated. When the clinical trials process was, for the most part, a small endeavor involving a limited number of investigators and sites, it made sense for investigators to turn to their patient populations for study candidates. With the dramatic growth in the industry, this traditional approach can no longer be relied on to produce the number of volunteers needed. A more professional solution is indicated, yet staff members responsible for this activity often have little or no training in recruitment techniques best suited for various therapeutic indications.

Training in patient recruitment techniques is a burgeoning industry. Today, there are recruitment providers, training companies and various associations accepting the challenge of training investigative sites on the ins and outs of recruitment. An important outcome of training may be that trained staff members are more likely to understand the federal regulations that apply to recruitment, and, therefore, may be more compliant. Training of this type can take place in the classroom, online, or at industry meetings, and, sometimes, may offer continuing education credits.

Increasingly, industry sponsors are recognizing the value of training CRAs in recruitment practices. They also prefer to select sites trained in patient recruitment. To enlarge the pool of trained sites, some sponsors are underwriting the cost of this training. This is an important step toward relationship building with sites that appreciate this training and are empowered by it. Those sites may feel an allegiance to the sponsors who invested in the training and may view them as a "preferred" sponsor when considering competitive assignments.

In the future, there may be a movement toward certifying sites that have received comprehensive training in patient recruitment. The specifics of this certification are unknown at the time of this writing, but perhaps they could follow the path of certification of study coordinators, study monitors and clinical investigators, which includes course work, an examination following a period of time on the job and continuing education.

Research organizations that implement recruitment SOPs and provide ongoing training build a strong foundation for the realization of best practices. Because these processes are so new, there are no industry-wide metrics, just anecdotal suggestions that training improves recruitment initiatives. The next horizon will be to document, through metrics, the increase in successful recruitment and retention campaigns. As metrics are developed over time, these best practices will take on a more evidence-based validity.

Key Takeaways

- A best practices working environment starts with the development, training and implementation of standard operating procedures (SOPs).
- Staff members must receive consistent messages that SOPs are guidelines with a purpose, not suggestions, and, therefore, must be followed.
- To encourage buy-in, it is a good idea to encourage discussion about the SOPs, to solicit input and to have a multi-person committee review the SOPs on a routine basis, such as annually.
- Training in patient recruitment is a best practice and is strongly needed by investigative sites to increase their skills in developing comprehensive recruitment campaigns.
- Training in patient recruitment should focus on a wide range of proactive strategies that address project feasibility, resource planning, return-on-investment (ROI) assessment, regulatory and ethical issues and media planning.
- Some sponsors are interested in underwriting training for sites in patient recruitment because they view this investment as key to enlarging the pool of better-trained sites.
- Because the implementation of best practices is a new concept for patient recruitment, there are few, if any, metrics documenting its success. Going forward, it is expected that a database of metrics will be established.

References

1. American Productivity and Quality Center, www.apqc.org/best, accessed September 11, 2003.
2. Siebel Systems, www.siebel.com/bestpractices/whatare.stm, accessed September 12, 2003.
3. American Productivity and Quality Center, www.apqc.org/portal/ apqc/site/generic?path=/site/benchmarking/overview.jhtml, accessed September 15, 2003.
4. Ibid., American Productivity and Quality Center.
5. *Standard Operating Procedures for Good Clinical Practice by Sponsors*, Center for Clinical Research Practice, Inc., Anna J. DeMarinis, et al., 2001.
6. *Recruiting Study Subjects*, FDA Information Sheets, www.fda.gov/oc/ ohrt/irbs/toc4.html#recruiting, accessed September 17, 2003.
7. CenterWatch, Boston, Mass., 2003.
8. *Vital Decisions: How Internet users decide what information to trust when they or loved ones are sick*, Pew Internet & American Life Project, May 2002. www.pewinternet.org/reports/pdfs/ PIP_Vital_Decisions_May2002.pdf.
9. "Improving Recruitment and Retention Practices Based on Input From the Public and Patients," CenterWatch, 2003.
10. *Protecting Personal Health Information in Research, Understanding the HIPAA Privacy Rule*, Department of Health and Human Services, http://privacyruleandresearch.nih.gov/pdf/HIPAA_Booklet_4-14-2003.pdf , accessed September 18, 2003.
11. *The Impact of HIPAA on Subject Recruitment in Clinical Trials*, Drug Information Association Conference, April 29, 2003, Carol A. Pratt, Ph.D., J.D.
12. "Improving Recruitment and Retention Practices Based on Input From the Public and Patients," CenterWatch, 2003.
13. *Selecting Investigators*, 21 Code of Federal Regulations Part 312.53(a).
14. *How to Grow Your Investigative Site*, Barry M. Miskin, M.D., and Ann Neuer, CenterWatch, 2002, p. 35.
15. The Management Assistance Program for Non-Profits, www.mapnp.org, accessed September 21, 2003.
16. CenterWatch, 2003.

Author Biographies

Diana L. Anderson, Ph.D.
President and CEO, D. L. Anderson International, Inc.
Dr. Diana L. Anderson is the President, CEO and Founder of D. L. Anderson International, Inc., parent company to subsidiaries D. Anderson &

Company, a patient recruitment provider and RRI, a Contract Research Organization. D. Anderson & Company, the patient recruitment arm of D. L. Anderson International, Inc., provides a comprehensive menu of specialized services to the clinical trials industry. These services include consulting and patient recruitment management, market research and feasibility assessments, media management and purchasing, creative development, regulatory management, clinical trial branding, community outreach and public relations, site-specific recruitment services, direct-to-consumer strategies, call center support and retention programs.

Dr. Anderson consults globally as a recognized authority in the field of patient recruitment, with recent presentations in Japan, Europe and Israel. She is widely published and frequently featured for her accomplishments in a variety of trade publications and scientific journals. She is also the author of the books *50 Ways to Cope with Arthritis, A Guide to Patient Recruitment* and *A Guide to Patient Recruitment and Retention.*

Dr. Anderson serves on several corporate boards and in various capacities on committees including Immediate Past Chair of the Association of Clinical Research Professionals (ACRP). She has previously held appointments on the Board of Directors of the North Texas Chapter of the Arthritis Foundation; Editorial Board, Arthritis Today Magazine; Past President, Association of Rheumatology Health Professionals (ARHP); Board of Trustees of the National Arthritis Foundation; Board of Directors, American College of Rheumatology; and Past President, Western U.S.A. Pain Society. She maintains memberships and remains actively involved in a number of these professional organizations.

She holds a Ph.D. from Texas Woman's University, M.S.N. from the University of Texas Health Care Science Center in San Antonio, Texas, and a B.S.N. from the University of Nebraska.

Nanette Myers, BS
Director of Patient Recruitment, D. Anderson & Company
Nanette Myers is the Director of Patient Recruitment for D. Anderson & Company (DAC), a multi-therapeutic patient recruitment provider. Myers manages all outsourcing vendors for DAC and administers the development and implementation of DAC's Standard Operating Procedures. In addition, she coordinates all ongoing patient recruitment campaigns. She specializes in the management of recruitment campaigns in the therapeutic areas of endocrinology, oncology and ophthalmology. Myers authored *Dry Eyes...Should You Be Concerned?* and has contributed to industry newsletters and publications. She is also an active member in the North Texas Association of Clinical Research Professionals (ACRP), serving as the newsletter co-chair.

Previously, Myers was a Sr. Regulatory Coordinator for US Oncology, Inc., the leading SMO in cancer research. She also holds a Bachelor of Science in Biomedical Science from Texas A&M University and is currently pursuing her MBA from the University of Texas at Dallas.

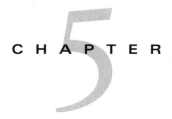

C H A P T E R

Decision-Making: Where Subject Recruitment and Ethics Meet

Matthew D. Whalen, Ph.D., President
Felix A. Khin-Maung-Gyi, Pharm.D., M.B.A., CIP, Chief Executive Officer
Chesapeake Research Review, Inc.

Objectives
- Define the three key challenges at play in recruiting and retaining subjects for clinical research studies.
- Identify and exemplify five ethical principles that are applicable to subject recruitment.
- Identify "executing" decision-making in subject recruitment.
- Demonstrate how ethical considerations are critical.

This chapter is not meant to be an exhaustive treatment of ethics and/or the regulations of biomedical and behavioral research; nor of subject recruitment. However, it is intended to raise awareness of their interaction and its importance. The reader is directed to other authoritative texts for more elaborate discussions on the history and principles of ethics, evolution of the regulations governing clinical research and informed consent concerns.[1-5]

Introduction

Societal awareness of issues in clinical research is often promoted as a result of crises, challenges or major events, whether domestically or internationally. Often, the development of applications of ethics is spurred on by these same events, either to assist in resolving the crisis or challenge or to strengthen national and international regulation.[6-11]

From the Nuremberg Code[12] to the Declaration of Helsinki,[13] to The Belmont Report,[14] to the guidelines from the Council for International Organizations of Medical Sciences (CIOMS),[15] what has come to be known as bioethics in biomedical research has been defined through principles.

Fundamental to the Nuremberg Code is the requirement of informed consent from potential subjects and the adequate evaluation of both the risks entailed as well as the science, in order to justify inclusion of human subjects, prior to their participation in research. In addition to consideration of clinical and scientific matters, the Declaration of Helsinki addresses the need for the research to be reviewed by an independent body. The Belmont Report, resulting from a National Commission's efforts, outlines basic principles of respect for individuals and articulates the need for the population bearing the risk(s) of participating in research to also enjoy the benefits of the findings.

It is primarily those sentinel documents that regulate authorizing the Institutional Review Board (IRB) as the governing entity overseeing the protection of the rights and welfare of human subjects participating in research. (21 Code of Federal Regulations, Part 56). Similarly, regulations governing the scope and content of informed consent (21 Code of Federal Regulations Part 50) were also generated based on these documents and principles within. (Noteworthy is the fact that while the regulations cited above relate to FDA-regulated products, there exist similar regulations for all federally funded research involving human subjects.)

Ethical Review Boards or Committees (ERBs or ERCs) and Institutional Review Boards (IRBs), collectively referred to here as IRBs, in compliance with governing regulations, apply those regulations and principles in making determinations related to protecting the rights and welfare of human subjects participating in a range of research activities.

In addition to sound clinical and scientific design of proposed research, key principles that have served as touchstones for all individuals involved in research include, for example, autonomy and permission. These principles emphasize freedom of individual choice and appropriate acknowledgment by an individual to participate in clinical research. They are the core of both being informed and giving consent. Complementing these principles are those of voluntary participation (that is, the subject does so without undue influence; or, more practically in today's healthcare environment, with minimal coercion).

Individual awareness, on the other hand, of the availability of a research study specific to the individual's therapeutic needs, is met through access to information directly or indirectly and actively or passively as provided by the researcher or their staff. Direct-to-consumer advertising, notices of ongoing research studies posted in clinics and referral (by lay personnel and professional staff) are examples. Such recruitment efforts for pharmaceutical company-sponsored studies recently have become more concerted, better coordinated and funded, in an attempt to enhance timely and efficient enrollment of subjects into clinical research studies.

Both HHS's Office for Human Research Protections (OHRP, formerly the Office of Protection from Research Risks, OPRR) and the FDA interpret[16] the use of such efforts to be the beginning of the informed consent process as well as study subject selection. As such, although specific and clear regulatory guidance remains nebulous at best, all forms of recruitment, direct advertisement in particular, are required to receive IRB review and approval prior to implementation and use.

Reports[17, 18] issued by the U.S. Office of the Inspector General (OIG) found that the system charged with protecting the rights and welfare of subjects is deficient in consistently applying ethical review and oversight of recruitment activities. The reports criticized the lack of regulatory will and direction in empowering IRBs to act with authority and consistency. The reports suggest that the lack of adequate oversight has resulted in improper subject identification, selection and inclusion into clinical studies with harm to some.

The volume and complexity of clinical research being conducted, fueled by rapidly advancing technology, continue to increase in response to market and public pressures. Equally significant is the public attention being drawn to clinical research by the popular press.

The challenge for all participants is juggling or balancing appreciation of regulations, law, well-constructed clinical science, and financial and economic pressures along with the practical necessities of conducting trials. The challenge is even greater because regulations, laws and ethical principles function similarly, and multi-dimensionally:

- they provide baselines, or the minimum requirements;
- they are highly subject to interpretation and application;
- they rely on interpretive bodies to determine precedents and rationale for decisions—many of which are subject to turnover; and,
- they are snapshots in time even when considering the exact same issues.

While charged with protecting the rights and welfare of human subjects, the IRB itself is not a patient advocacy body (i.e., advocate for a specific therapeutic area such as cancer); nor is it a judiciary entity; nor a scientific peer review committee in a strict definition; nor an instrument of public policy; nor a regulatory affairs department; nor an ethics committee. Yet, it must take into account these various and variant concerns and apply all those perspectives when debating subject protection issues for any given research project.

For better or for worse, the challenge of juggling and balancing is one quite familiar for IRBs.

Subject Recruitment

Ethical and regulatory interpretation assumes recruitment of subjects as the beginning of the informed consent process engaging/inviting potential subjects to participate in the research.

Research and practice may be, and often are, carried on together around the world. However, a critical distinction is the goal: for research, clean data; for practice, therapy. Subject recruitment efforts need to clearly communicate this difference so as not to mislead potential subjects. Therapy may or may not be a fortuitous effect of the research. This is particularly true in early Phase trials and in any research with the possibility of "therapeutic misconception."

Traditionally, regulatory attention and the IRB practice of providing oversight of recruitment programs have been largely targeted at the direct advertising to patients with the indication being studied. However, three realities pervade recruitment as it is now practiced:

- Subjects can either be viewed as commodities or as offering a gift of themselves;
- Recruitment includes retention in order to achieve the primary goal of clinical research: clean data; and,
- Recruitment and retention pose a significant threat to achieving "quality speed."

Ample evidence abounds that each is instrumental in designing, developing and implementing recruitment campaigns.

In the brave new world of global clinical research, marketing, public relations, advertising and technology have had a marked impact on subject recruitment, especially as they are systemically integrated to create a recruitment and retention campaign. Elaborate campaigns—both in depth and scope—have been developed for trials in virtually all therapeutic areas and all phases. Recruitment practices commonly employed today are often combined and include, among others: direct advertising to the subject population; incentives to physicians, other caregivers or family and friends to refer potential subjects to researchers; incentives to researchers and their staff to enhance enrollment of subjects; identification of potential study candidates from the physician/caregiver database(s); and identification of eligibility of patients through medical record/ancillary report review. Initiatives to keep subjects in the study, once enrolled, or "fulfillment programs," are an extension of the recruitment process.

Ethical Issues in Subject Recruitment

Illustrations of ethically loaded questions are: Why is advertising to potential subjects bad? Shouldn't patients be told of research that might be of benefit to them? How is advertising of research any different than any other type of advertising? If a patient were referred to another physician for participation in a research study, wouldn't the physicians have the patient's best interest in mind before suggesting enrollment in a study?

Different phases of drug development research and different biomedical and behavioral research processes have different ethical issues. Recruiting subjects, therefore, confronts ethical issues associated both with study start-up and with different phases. The principle that appears to be violated when potential subjects enter studies based on misinformation, intentional or inadvertent, is undue influence.

Undue Influence and Coercion

From the vantage of an IRB, it is charged with reviewing and approving any information that a potential subject comes in contact with relating to a specific clinical trial as part of recruitment. That information includes the whole media of recruitment (including graphics, music, text, layout, format and so on). After all, again, the material and campaign are also the beginning of the informed consent process: the first opportunity the potential subject has to begin to become informed about a trial.

Hence, being informed, or misled, is a process beginning with that information.

This reality places significant restraints on the creativity of public relations, media and advertising professionals, recognizing that the goal of such professionals is to convince the buyer to agree to the message. What IRBs as well as sponsors and site personnel must separate is information from misinformation. Suspending disbelief is useful in assuming that the intention is not to: mislead; suggest that participating in research is better in some shape or form than standard care; imply that the research is "new and improved" compared to standard therapies; or overly promise financial or other therapeutic incentives for participation.

As the clinical research enterprise becomes more competitive and, with the assistance of mass media, the realities and perception of fraud increases, it is ethically incumbent upon those participating in research to examine what other types of fraud can exist beyond that of illegal handling of revenues or misappropriation of pharmaceuticals. In brief: the information and messages of recruitment campaigns can be unduly influential, not simply somewhat persuasive. And an equally important issue is the public perception that those behind the message are participants in fraud.

A more obvious aspect of undue influence involves inducements to participate or continue in the study. Ethicists try to distinguish this by dubbing it "coercion." Inappropriate inducements may be offered to the subject, investigator and investigator's staff, colleagues who refer patients to participate or to the potential subject's friends or family. While the potential harm to subjects being coerced to remain in the study for reasons solely due to receiving monetary or other inducements is readily evident, less obvious is the involvement of healthcare professionals. There exists a prevailing concern that incentives to physicians to refer patients or to investigators to accelerate enrollment are a conflict of interest, not to mention potential violations of local laws, regulations and medical codes of conduct.

Each IRB makes its own judgments in the area of payment to/for subjects participating in clinical research trials. Their basis for decisions is the principle of distributive justice (from the Belmont Report and other documents on research ethics) and avoidance of unacceptable inducements for subject participation (e.g., lack of coercion). While the U.S. regulations are silent on this issue, the "Canadian Tri-Council Policy Statement in Ethical Conduct for Research Involving Humans" provides some guidance for IRBs from the perspective of a proportionate approach in reviewing the incentives and conflicts of interest. That document suggests that the IRB evaluate the nature of the conflict of interest and make a subjective determination of relative magnitude. So, if the IRB perceives the conflict to be relatively small, the investigator is asked to disclose this conflict. The investigator, however, would be asked to abandon involvement if the conflict is determined by the IRB to be significant.

An IRB does consider other factors in its deliberations about whether a proposed payment for a clinical trial subject is reasonable. The factors may vary depending on the project being considered, and not all are applicable in every instance. The deliberation of such factors is, again, driven by reference to ethical principles, as well as practical understanding of the clinical research process and regulatory requirements and guidelines.

These factors include the purpose of the payment (for example: acknowledging the altruistic participation of the subject, thanking a person; reimbursement for an expense; compensation for time or lost wages; or compensation for a subject's efforts or pain because of research procedures). They also include the level of risk compared to benefit; as well as factors related to the autonomy of the subject (for example: age, dependent relationship with study staff, the person's economic status, among others).

Other factors include the nature of the payment (cash, cash-equivalent, an object of value; as well as the impact of the payment as it may be related to privacy or confidentiality, such as the necessity of reporting earnings to the IRS or other federal, state and local authorities).

Access to healthcare itself is an inducement to participate in research. This is especially true in economically disadvantaged countries and communities, and in circumstances of disease states for which there are no, or not enough, viable alternatives. To avoid real or perceived conflicts and issues of coercion, IRB deliberation includes not only the matter of payment to subjects but also other inducements to participate.

Equitability is yet another factor of concern, raising questions such as: what is the range of variation of compensation among sites in a multi-site study; how wide is the range; what accounts for the range; is there a potential bias for/against inclusion of certain subjects; and how do community attitudes and local conditions impact the types and amounts of compensation offered in one area versus another?

As an aside, if a physician practice simply wishes to announce participation in clinical research, as a broad announcement, such promotion does not require IRB review and approval. Information associated with a specific study, however, does require IRB review and approval. Hence, the IRB's purview with respect to screening potential subjects includes review of everything from scripts used by call center interviewers to simple flyers tacked onto walls of clinics.

Screening Subjects & Confidentiality and Privacy

Identification of eligible subjects, in addition to the recruitment processes mentioned above, may include review of existing databases correlating inclusion and exclusion criteria to patient medical histories and demographics. Historically, only the patient's physician and caregiver evaluated patients in physician practices. The mounting economic pressures on physicians and clinical researchers to remain competitive have resulted in exploration of the use of patient profiles in an attempt to accelerate enrollment.

More efficient screening of potential subjects is a crucial element of recruitment and retention efforts. Hence, systematic attention has been focused on this facet of the clinical research process; so much so that a burgeoning sub-industry has grown up around the screening process. Dampening enthusiasm, however, is HIPAA, the lack of regulatory clarifying guidance, and, as a result, a potentially conservative posture among IRBs (that is, when the regulations are silent, IRBs exist to manage risk following what makes reasonable ethical sense). With heightened awareness about the privacy of health information and confidentiality of the patient/subject-physician/staff relationship, technology-assisted solutions to recruitment and screening need to be carefully assessed.

Faced with the twin threats of regulatory and legal sanction, the clinical research enterprise has been somewhat hampered in its efforts to recruit more efficiently. The ethical dimension of the matter, however, has less to do with individual freedom and more to do with informed consent and permission.

Simply stated, patient records should not be reviewed for research-related activities without prior permission from the patient or legally authorized representative. Similarly, following obtaining consent from the patient, mechanisms should exist to enable the patient to withdraw consent at any time without jeopardizing any of the benefits to which the patient is otherwise entitled. A key mechanism is the ability to identify those who have given consent should they rescind it, or, request that they not be contacted for research-related activities. It should be inherent to any process where database screening is considered.

Two final points:

- With or without technology, there is no such thing as complete privacy or confidentiality; and to convey otherwise is disingenuous, if not unethical.
- Working with technology transforms the issue of confidentiality and privacy to one of security in no small measure. As a result, even the methods of technology come under the purview of ethical review.

Summary

The fact that IRBs are overburdened to meet today's burgeoning demands of the clinical research enterprise is well known and accepted. While regulatory review is assigned to the IRB, it would be counterproductive to place the burden of oversight regarding the protection of the rights and welfare of human subjects solely on one part of the clinical research enterprise.

The movement toward accreditation of Human Research Protections Programs reinforces the shared responsibilities of sponsor, site, IRB and subject. Ethics training, as part of certification of professionals or separate from it, does as well.

Table 1: Relationships Involved/Affected by the Research Process

Not only from an ethical perspective but also from that of practicality, trust is the underpinning of the clinical research enterprise:

- patients' trust in care providers and caregivers;
- trust of volunteers founded in the assumption that researchers will adhere to the highest principles of clinical and scientific care in conducting the research;
- researchers' trust that the sponsor of the research will utilize the information collected from subjects in good faith in an appropriate manner, applying the highest standards;
- sponsors' trust that the researchers have the core competencies necessary to collect clean data in a timely manner; and,
- regulatory agencies' trust that all participants in the research process will abide by all applicable regulations.

Table 1 illustrates the relationship between all those involved/affected by the research process. Violation of trust by any of the participants in the scheme results in tremendously negative results. Many times it is easy to place the blame of wrongdoings on another party. However, it is incumbent on each of us not to violate that trust ultimately given to us by the subject.

Key Takeaways

- Informed consent begins with recruitment activities.
- There are three guiding ethical principles behind decision-making in clinical research that are also the basis of regulations. They are Beneficence, Justice and Respect for Persons, as articulated in the Belmont Report.
- Issues of privacy and coercion point out most dramatically the importance of decision-making at the intersection of ethics and subject recruitment. The goal of all privacy law is to maximize the power of individual decision at the source of the information at risk.
- The more ethical principles are considered and used to develop and drive public understanding and the use of technology, the better the chances for more thorough-going acceptance of clinical research as a whole.
- Ethics is no longer the privileged domain of a few academicians. It is now the responsibility of all of us in clinical research.

Appendix I

Practical Guidelines

The following are suggestions that may provide a practical approach to recruitment issues:

Recruiting Subjects: Advertisements, Flyers, Letters

A very simple, short "notice" format is appropriate. It should contain: that you are conducting a research study and a brief objective of the study; what drug/device/biologics is involved (and/or therapeutic area involved); general description of subjects to be enrolled; and a contact person. Subsequent direct screening during enrollment of subjects will give subjects the opportunity to get additional information and to ask any questions to clarify information in the short notice.

For more elaborate recruitment notices, the following may assist in order to meet the spirit and letter of federal government regulations:

- This is a research study in which you/your organization, by name, is participating.
- What exactly is being studied that impacts the individual subject.
- The duration of the study and what is expected of the individual subject. For example, the number of visits to your facility in the

course of the study, and what the subject must do, such as keep a diary or use a drug or device.

- The benefits that the subject will receive only as directly related to the study: for example, free study-related drug/device/biologics, free study-related tests (and what kinds), free study-related examinations (and what kinds).

- Monetary compensation—separate from benefits—that the enrolled subject may expect to receive, including travel expense reimbursement.

- A statement that includes, "If you or someone you know is interested in participating, please contact…," and indicate an individual and his/her phone number.

- The name of a specific person who may be the Principal Investigator, the Research Coordinator or a designated staff member of your organization or practice.

- Use of "research" or "investigational" as descriptors rather than words like "new" (or any similar term suggesting "improved" or "better" or "different therefore having more advantage").

- If the recruitment material includes graphics: Look carefully at any illustrations in the literature to assure they are appropriate to the subject population being studied (in terms of gender, ethnicity, age, for example) and that the illustrations are inclusive of the diversity of the population that is being recruited. This is particularly true for human representations.

- Note also that typefaces used and size need to be carefully considered so that they do not constitute misleading enticements; as might the overemphasized use of the word "free."

- Avoid language that focuses on your site, your organization or your reputation as opposed to what subjects need to know—words like: "the largest," "most experienced" and "leading expert"—or words and phrases that suggest the same thing.

- Specifically regarding indications of benefits, suggestion of coercion is a critical concern.

Recruiting Subjects: Using Audio and/or Visual Media

All the suggestions made that apply to print materials also apply to audio and visual presentations, especially those relating to graphics. In audio and visual presentations, the same sensitivity can be shown in selecting appropriate voices, actors or dynamic images.

Making such selections means balancing what might appeal to the populations particularly targeted for the study with the regulatory guidelines relating to inclusion of minority and women populations. Additional appreciation needs to be considered if special populations are being recruited (such as children, physically or mentally challenged, institutionalized individuals, among others).

Another dimension of audio and visual presentations are the stagings and settings. Dramatic images, or sounds, that suggest a level of competency, trust or credibility that is not accurate to the study or study site being advertised can be coercive. For example:

- A video presentation using settings or scenes which display large complexes of buildings or equipment to suggest an excellence of facilities that in fact will not be used;
- A sound-/look-alike actor with resemblance to a trusted authority in a specific community, or in society, used in a manner that is not highly obviously humorous;
- A web site with graphics and interactivity highly appealing to a particular population that also emphasizes financial compensation and/or suggests that being a "professional subject" is a viable means of making a living.

The fundamental approach is to keep the advertising piece clear, simple and accurate. Neither the FDA nor the IRB is looking for award-winning creativity, which might be construed to be coercive.

Database

The screening process for enrollment of subjects subsequent to their recruitment gives the study coordinator another opportunity to get additional information from the prospective subjects in order to develop a database assuring that all appropriate populations have access to participation.

In developing site databases of any kind, including adoption of already created practice systems, it is critical to build in confidentiality protection for each subject or applicant. Requirements of the sponsor organization may or may not be sufficient from regulatory, legal or ethical perspectives, since the sponsor does not necessarily have either complete access to the systems or the right to protect them.

One way to anticipate potential issues concerning inclusion, access and confidentiality is to plan the study anticipating that the following questions can be answered with "YES" (that is, ways in which something might have been done better) after the study is over:

- Could you tell that the study population described in the protocol fairly reflects the eligible population in clinical practice by: (a) age; (b) gender; (c) ethnicity?
- If you used multiple sites, is the above still true?
- Could you access this type of information in a way that provides general results only or in a coded fashion, preventing correlation of this information with the name of the subject?
- Were there conditions of the study excluding certain populations: for example, the number of visits to your facility in the course of the study (issue of subjects' access to transportation); and what the subject must do, such as keep a diary or use a drug or device (issue of subjects' literacy or innumeracy capability)?

- Were financial benefits realized appropriately—that is, involving balancing short-term discomforts, indignities, risks with longer-term gains and risks for the use of the subject's body?
- Were the subjects enrolling in the study primarily for the financial benefits they gained? (Issue here, appreciating that "how much is too much" is circumstantial: the benefit to the subjects are financial to such a degree that discomforts, indignities or risks they might otherwise not assume are temporarily ignored by subjects at the risk of physical and/or emotional harm.)

References

1. Engelhardt HT. *The Foundation of Bioethics.* New York, NY: Oxford University Press; 1996.
2. Beauchamp TL, Childress J. *Principles of Biomedical Ethics.* New York, NY; Oxford University Press; 1996.
3. Levine RJ. *Ethics and Regulation of Clinical Research.* New Haven, CT: Yale University Press; 1988.
4. Grisso T, Applebaum PS. *Assessing Competence to Consent to Treatment.* New York, NY; Oxford University Press; 1998.
5. Hartnett T, editor. *The Complete Guide to Informed Consent in Clinical Trials.* PharmSource Information Services, 2000.
6. Epstein KC, Sloat B. "Drug Trials: Do People Know the Truth about Experiments? In the Name of Healing." Cleveland, OH: *The Plain Dealer*; December 15, 1996.
7. Sloat B, Epstein KC. "Drug Trials: Do People Know the Truth about Experiments? Using Our Kids as Guinea Pigs." Cleveland, OH: *The Plain Dealer*; December 16, 1996.
8. Epstein KC, Sloat B. "Drug Trials: Do People Know the Truth about Experiments? Foreign Tests Don't Meet U.S. Criteria." Cleveland, OH: *The Plain Dealer*; December 17, 1996.
9. Sloat B, Epstein KC. "Drug Trials: Do People Know the Truth about Experiments? Overseers Operate in the Dark." Cleveland, OH: *The Plain Dealer*; December 18, 1996.
10. Weiss R, Nelson D. U.S. Halts Cancer Tests in Oklahoma. Washington, DC: *The Washington Post*; July 11, 2000.
11. Weiss R, Nelson D. FDA Faults Penn Animal Tests That Led to Fatal Human Trial; Genetic Research Killed Teenager. Washington, DC: *The Washington Post*; July 12, 2000.
12. The Nuremberg Code. *JAMA.* 1996;276:1691.
13. World Medical Association Declaration of Helsinki: Recommendations Guiding Medical Doctors in Biomedical Research Involving Human Subjects. Adopted by the 18th World Medical Assembly, Helsinki, Finland, June 1964 and amended by the 29th World Medical Assembly,

Tokyo, Japan, October 1975, 35th World Medical Assembly, Venice, Italy, October 1983, 41st World Medical Assembly, Hong Kong, September 1989, and the 48th General Assembly, Somerset West, Republic of South Africa, October 1996.

14. National Commission for the Protection of Human Subjects. The Belmont Report. Washington, DC: US Government Printing Office; 1979.

15. Council for the International Organizations of Medical Sciences. International Ethical Guidelines for Biomedical Research Involving Human Subjects. Geneva, Switzerland: CIOMS; 1993.

16. FDA Information Sheets. *Guidance for Institutional Review Boards and Clinical Investigators*. Rockville, MD: 1998.

17. Office of Inspector General. *Recruiting Human Subjects: Pressures in Industry-Sponsored Clinical Research*. www.dhs.gov/progorg/oei. June 2000.

18. Office of Inspector General. *Recruiting Human Subjects: Sample Guidelines for Practice*. www.dhs.gov/progorg/oei. June 2000.

Author Biographies

Matthew D. Whalen, Ph.D.
President, Co-Founder, Chesapeake Research Review, Inc.
Dr. Whalen co-founded and co-leads Chesapeake Research Review, Inc., a company named to the Fast 50 or Fast 500 (a program Sponsored by Deloitte & Touche) four times that has also received the Blue Chip Enterprise Award (Sponsored by the U.S. Chamber of Commerce).

He has over twenty years experience advising on managing organization and work unit change in start-up through mature organizations. He has facilitated professional development sessions for industry, government, academic, non-profit and multi-lateral executives and senior managers; as well as provided private coaching.

Immediately prior to Chesapeake Research Review, Inc., Whalen served as a Vice President of the Washington, DC, region of an international management consulting firm. Clients included Forbes and Inc. 500 companies, federal agencies and trade associations. Earlier, he ran the office of a national consulting firm, directing a company-wide task force reorganizing services and functions.

He had also been active in economic development, coordinating two industry/government partnerships, winning a U.S. Presidential Citation. As an expert on workplace trends, he has been quoted in media ranging from *Executive Update* and *New Woman* to *Money, USA Today* and *Reader's Digest*.

Throughout his professional career, he has been a faculty member at institutions including Temple University, Trinity College, and University of

Maryland in areas ranging from business and public policy to science, technology and society.

He is a frequent chair, speaker, moderator or panelist at national and regional industry and professional conferences, particularly on issues integrating clinical research, public policy, social issues and ethics.

He serves on the Editorial Boards of *Clinical Researcher* and *Journal of GxP Compliance*. He is co-author of the following publications: "Electronic Data Capture Issues for IRBs: Administrative and Regulatory" in *DIA Journal*; and the "Ethical and Confidentiality-Based Issues in Patient Recruitment Today" chapter in *A Guide to Patient Recruitment: Today's Best Practices and Proven Strategies* (2001). He has also contributed to *The Complete Guide to Informed Consent in Clinical Trials* (2000).

His Ph.D. focus was science, technology and society (University of Maryland, College Park). Post-graduate work included mediation (University of Vermont), organization development (Georgetown University) and bioethics (National Institutes of Health).

Felix A. Khin-Maung-Gyi, Pharm.D., M.B.A., CIP
CEO, Founder, Chesapeake Research Review, Inc.

In addition to heading Chesapeake Research Review, Inc., in early 2003, Dr. Gyi was appointed to the U.S. Secretary of Health and Human Services' Human Research Protections Advisory Committee (SACHRP). He is also currently doing research, as a Senior Policy Fellow with the Center for Drugs and Public Policy, University of Maryland, on the interplay of ethics, public policy and economics; and conjointly serving as Visiting Research Assistant Professor in the Department of Pharmacy Practice and Science of the same institution.

Internationally, Dr. Khin-Maung-Gyi has been asked to advise the Ministry of Health of the Union of Myanmar (Burma) in Yangon to explore the further development of biomedical research, including education and training in research ethics in that country. In 2002, at the invitation of the U.S. Department of Health and Human Services and the International Science and Technology Council, Dr. Khin-Maung-Gyi, Dr. Whalen and other colleagues provided clinical research operations and ethics consultation to research institutes from Russia, Georgia and Kazakhstan.

Overall, for twenty years, Dr. Khin-Maung-Gyi has provided consultation and professional development as well as managed research units, IRBs and projects in both private and academic sectors. He has worked internationally, traveling and living abroad as well. Throughout his professional career, Dr. Khin-Maung-Gyi has also served on university faculty.

He is a frequent chair, speaker, moderator or panelist at forums ranging from national professional conferences to Investigator Meetings. Dr. Khin-Maung-Gyi is co-author of the book *Ethics of the Use of Human Subjects in Research* and chapters in other books as well as articles in such publications as *DIA Journal* and *Applied Clinical Trials*. He serves as an Editorial Advisor of the Clinical Trials Advisor and of the Association for Clinical Research

Professionals' (ACRP) journal, *The Monitor*. He has been the subject of a recent interview in *Clinical Researcher*.

Dr. Khin-Maung-Gyi received his Doctor of Pharmacy degree from Duquesne University and his M.B.A. (Executive Program) from Loyola (MD) College. He has completed clinical pharmacy residencies in both pediatric and adult medicine and done post-graduate studies in bioethics, drug development, regulations and medical research. His undergraduate work in pharmacy included a concentration in microbiology.

PART TWO

Implementation
and
Process

C H A P T E R

The Patient Recruitment Process: A Science and an Art

Diana L. Anderson, Ph.D., D. Anderson & Company

Objectives

- Describe how scientific and artistic principles apply to the patient recruitment process
- Discuss growing use of informatics, a scientific, evidence-based method for site selection and investigator selection
- Highlight the value of early planning as a technique with promise for meeting enrollment targets on time and within budget
- Spot a trend toward greater collaboration among recruitment providers
- Discuss the emergence of patient recruitment forums and associations within the patient recruitment industry

Introduction

A new multi-center phase III osteoporosis study is about to begin across the United States. The sponsor is in the process of selecting eighty investigative sites, with an enrollment target of twenty-five volunteers for each site. At the end of the selection process, the site selector has chosen a mix of sites with varied experience in conducting osteoporosis studies. For some, this new trial does not seem substantially different from the ten osteoporosis trials they have conducted in the recent past. For other sites, osteoporosis is a fairly new therapeutic area and is one in which they are looking to expand their service offerings. Whether the site is experienced in osteoporosis studies, or just getting started, it will be expected to reach its enrollment goal.

How this hypothetical sponsor and the eighty sites go about meeting the enrollment targets underscores how the recruitment process is evolving toward greater sophistication. Sponsors, investigative sites and recruitment providers are introducing elements of art and science into their planning strategies. Metrics are being used increasingly to document success of various recruitment initiatives, such as site selection and media choices, for the recruitment campaign. Recruitment providers are starting to collaborate to offer a comprehensive array of recruitment services. The investigator meeting may become a forum for soliciting investigator opinion about the structure of recruitment campaigns. A look at changing recruitment practices and processes is the subject of this chapter.

A Science and an Art

Recruitment processes are becoming more professional and systematic as they incorporate elements of scientific and artistic discipline. The intricate balance between the two is basic to the practice of medicine, and to the related field of clinical trials, which includes patient recruitment. In exploring how science and art complement each other in the context of patient recruitment, it is useful to establish working definitions of both.

Science can be defined as the observation, identification, description, experimental investigation and theoretical explanation of phenomena.[1,2] Science is deeply rooted in a scientific method designed to test a hypothesis, measure results from the testing, and ultimately drawing a conclusion (see Table 1). Experiments should also be reproducible by other experimenters to establish validity.

Table 1: The Scientific Method

- Observe and describe a phenomenon or group of phenomena
- Formulate a hypothesis to explain the phenomena
- Use the hypothesis to predict the existence of other phenomena, or to predict quantitatively the results of new observations (deductive reasoning)
- Perform experiments to test the predictions, and collect and analyze data, possibly resulting in modifying hypothesis and retesting it
- Derive conclusion

Source: www.journaloftheoretics.com/Editorials/Vol-1/e1-3.htm

---

Art has many definitions reflecting the broad-based use of the term. Fine and performing arts may be regarded as the conscious production or arrangement of sounds, colors, forms, movements or other elements in a manner that affects the sense of beauty.[3] Art is also defined as a system of principles and methods employed in the performance of a set of activities,[4] such as the *art* of public speaking, or the *art* of negotiation.

These definitions hint at the close relationship between science and art. When a scientist constructs a theory or hypothesis, this is an intuitive act that parallels the creative process of the artist.[5] When an artist lays out a painting, or when a speaker crafts a lecture, there are logical, scientific-type steps that are tried and often modified to determine flow and maximize impact.

In making a diagnosis, a physician evaluates and measures physical factors and symptoms, while also using his or her instincts about the patient's condition, based on experience and observation. In the related area of clinical development, aspects of science and art apply to the complexities of developing an investigational compound or device. There's the drafting of the protocol based on a hypothesis; selection of sites, often based on past experience; creation of case report forms; the collection, forwarding and analyzing of data generated by the studies; and amendments to protocols based on those data, to name a few of the many steps. And there is patient recruitment.

More of a Science

Making patient recruitment successful entails elements of science and art, perhaps with a bias toward the scientific. This bias reflects the growing recognition by clinical partners that recruitment is a complex endeavor, is often behind schedule[6] and could benefit from a methodical scientific approach to make measurable improvements.

Len Rosenberg, Ph.D., R.Ph., Managing Partner of eP2Consulting, a consulting firm offering technology and process solutions for drug development, sees patient recruitment activities as decidedly scientific. He says, "Our discipline is scientific in its very foundation. The process has end-points, data analysis, and objective measurement of patient progress. It's clear to me that successful patient recruitment comes down to precedents, principles and best practices that have worked. You always have to work with data and metrics to identify where the patients are. While there is a creative part involved in reaching prospects by developing certain messages that maximize response, you first have to look at the metrics and the discipline before you go to the art side. There is very little room for gut-feeling or seat-of-the-pants in the way you approach recruitment."

Gregg Sweet, Vice President of Integrated Clinical Trial Services, LLC, a patient recruitment provider, holds a similar opinion. Sweet comments, "You have to be open-minded enough to come up with creative new solutions, but for the most part, recruitment is a very scientific process. Ten years ago, the first central campaigns used mostly mass media, but ten years later, we use a huge toolbox for patient recruitment and enrollment. There is a science in knowing which tools to use, and in the required metrics to back up those decisions."

Table 2: Some Informatics Providers with Patient Recruitment Services

- Acurian
- ePharmaLearning
- Medstat (Division of Thomson Corp.)
- PharMetrics
- Verispan

Source: www.journaloftheoretics.com/Editorials/Vol-1/e1-3.htm

Evidence is accruing that science is playing an expanding role in the development of recruitment campaigns. For starters, there are companies and departments within companies dedicated to providing informatics services. Informatics, the science of using technology solutions to integrate, organize, analyze, manage and use information,[7] is growing within the clinical trials industry for applications linked to accelerating product development. Some providers are offering informatics services specific to patient recruitment (see Table 2), such as locating the needed study subjects, the right investigators and the right sites.

Table 3: Evidence-Based Site Selection

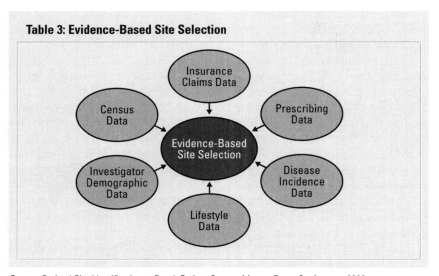

Source: Optimal Site Identification to Reach Patient Groups, Marcus Evans Conference, 2003

"More and more sponsors understand the interface between patient recruitment and site selection, and are starting to realize that selecting the right sites is 90% of successful patient recruitment", says Beth Harper, Senior Vice President of RRI International, Inc. According to Harper, sponsors are recognizing that the site selection process should be a scientific, evidence-based activity that relies on informatics tools such as disease incidence databases, insurance claims databases, prescribing databases, and more (see Table 3) to pinpoint the right sites and investigators.

Using databases and mapping techniques, informatics providers enable research organizations to identify geographical areas with high prevalence of the disease in question, and within those areas, zone in on practitioners in the top two or three deciles based on diagnostic code, prescribing habits and number of patient visits. Some of those practitioners may be clinical investigators. If not, mapping can identify the nearest investigator and the high volume practitioners within a five, ten, or twenty miles radius of that investigator (see Table 4). Using this methodical approach to finding the right physicians is important for predicting recruitment success because data suggest that physicians with higher numbers of office visits for specific diagnostic codes recruit more patients.

Table 4: Estimate Office Visits for Osteoarthritis in Philadelphia (Adults Aged 18 and Over)

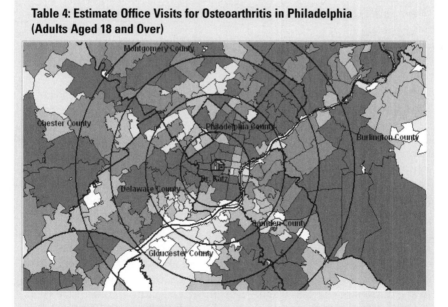

The investigator has good access to patients based on being in the highest (darkest) office visit area for osteoarthritis. The closest area, within the five-mile radius circle, is especially good.

Source: Optimal Site Identification to Reach Patient Groups, Marcus Evans Conference, 2003

The Science of Early Planning

Investigative sites participating in the hypothetical osteoporosis study described at the beginning of the chapter will benefit from early planning, one of the more progressive and scientifically based recruitment techniques. Early planning is about the sponsor tagging patient recruitment as a key component in the success of a multi-site clinical trial program, and taking specific steps—early on—to plan for success. This method starts with the sponsor establishing criteria for choosing the right recruitment provider to develop and implement the right plan of action from the very beginning (see Table 5). The sponsor might consider using a template for the request-for-proposal (RFP), enabling providers to prepare bids based on the same parameters.

Table 5: Selecting the Right Recruitment Provider for Early Planning Program

- Prior Experience
- Expertise
- Proven Track Record
- Cost
- Quality of Proposal
- Reporting Tools
- Available Resources
- Meet Turnaround Date for RFP

Source: D. Anderson & Co. and eP2Consulting, 2003

Early planning calls for the sponsor and selected recruitment provider to have strong interaction with the sites by soliciting their input on recruitment options specific to their sites. The results of this interactive approach are tallied and used to make some site-specific decisions about the central recruitment campaign. The expectation is that when sponsors and recruitment providers take site concerns into consideration and act on that information—there will be greater buy-in by sites and, hopefully, greater recruitment success. This proactive strategy is a marked departure from the sponsor's traditionally passive view of patient recruitment as just another expense or the responsibility of the sites, to be addressed later, after the investigator meeting or site initiation, or when lagging recruitment falls into rescue mode.

The value of early planning was illustrated in a multi-center diabetes study involving 75 sites. For this study, a national recruitment provider was selected, and together with the sponsor, an early action plan was crafted and rolled out in three ways: live participation at the investigators' meeting, live participation via webcast and viewing of the taped session of the investigators' meeting prior to site initiation.

As part of the presentation, a series of questions were posed to the investigators through personal digital assistants (PDAs). These questions asked investigators if advertising and outreach campaigns would be required and, if so, to state their preferences for certain media options. They were asked about willingness to participate in a centralized recruiting initiative, and more (see Table 6).

Table 6: Some Questions Asked of Investigators to Plan Patient Recruitment Campaign

- Whether the private practice can generate enough patients to meet enrollment objectives or if advertising and outreach programs would be required

- Willingness to participate in a centralized recruitment initiative, and the desired number of pre-screened patients to be referred to site

- Preferred types of community outreach (TV, radio, newspaper, Internet, etc.)

- Willingness to commit to a timeframe to contact pre-screened subjects for scheduling first appointment, i.e., same day, two days, etc.

Source: D. Anderson & Co. and eP2Consulting, 2003

Once results were tallied and analyzed, it became clear that there was diverse opinion as to what each site needed and wanted (see Table 7). With these data, outreach programs for the investigative sites could be customized, implemented and then adjusted, as indicated by metrics. Importantly, sites were made to feel that their input was needed and valued, so consequently they had more of a stake in making the program a success.

Table 7: What Is Your Preference for How Recruitment Support Should Be Handled?

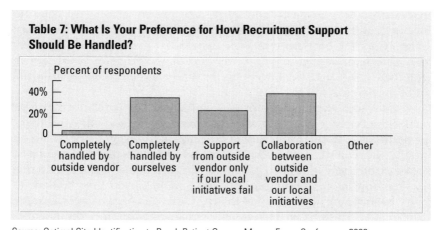

Source: Optimal Site Identification to Reach Patient Groups, Marcus Evans Conference, 2003

In the end, recruitment finished three weeks ahead of schedule, and within budget.

Bret Berner, Ph.D., Vice President Product Development at Depomed, Inc., a specialty pharmaceutical company, is a strong supporter of early planning for patient recruitment. "It's the best way I know of to begin and end a trial on time," Berner states.

The savings possible with early planning can be substantial. There are certain monthly costs to manage a trial, which are manifested either as fees paid to CROs to run the trial, or as expenses to internal budgets. When a study is completed on time, those monthly fees are no longer generated, representing a real savings to the sponsor. And as Berner points out, when the enrollment process is on schedule, the sponsor and CRO do not have to incur the expense of adding additional sites.

The Artistic Side of Patient Recruitment

In 2002, Robert Lull, M.D., then president of the San Francisco Medical Society, published a commentary in *San Francisco Medicine*, the organization's monthly magazine. Entitled *Balancing the Science and Art of Medicine*,[10] Lull's commentary discusses the profession's increasing reliance on evidence-based medicine as the exclusive focus for all patient care decisions. In an evidence-based mode, Lull writes, all diagnostic approaches and therapeutic plans must be based on scientifically valid peer-reviewed published literature. The evidence-based approach de-emphasizes intuition and unsystematic clinical experience as sufficient grounds for clinical decision-making.[11]

"I am a strong supporter of a scientific approach to medical decision-making, but I am concerned about overemphasis on this formalized approach," Lull says in the article. "Evidence-based medicine is clearly on the science side of medicine and spirituality falls on the art side. They are inherently different, almost opposites, yet both are powerful and necessary components for physicians in their approach to patient care. The best physicians have learned to balance the hard-nosed evidence-based science with their spiritual-based power of observation and intuition…This is the art of medicine."[12]

Experienced recruitment providers and others with patient recruitment responsibilities have long acknowledged that scientific and artistic skill sets are needed to craft successful patient recruitment campaigns. The science of locating the right sites is rooted in databases and metrics that document past successes, but there is more to patient recruitment than pouring over statistics. There are intangible components, with a more artistic turn. "You can do all of the mapping needed to find the right investigators and feel confident that your evidence-based recruitment initiatives will target the required audience, and identify the right mix of media tools, but the art is in getting the message right," says Beth Harper.

Hard data may clearly indicate that a recruitment campaign in one city should include advertisements on the local cable television station, an easy-listening radio station, health fairs, and direct mail. In another city, that same study may call for advertisements placed on the local country-western station, educational lectures at the local senior center and brochures for the local physicians' offices. Yet, despite this degree of specificity, without the right message, a recruitment campaign may be less than successful.

Crafting the right message is, indeed, an art. It has to reach the appropriate audience by appreciating their needs, interests and motivations. The message has to be understandable, interesting, eye-catching, ear-catching and have emotional appeal, creating a call to action, yet be conservative enough to be approved by an institutional review board (IRB) (see Table 8). "There is a way to do this and it takes an even more adept person to be creative in a controlled manner," Harper says.

Table 8: The Message

Message	How message relates to potential motivations of a study participant
Dry Eyes? Looking for a Solution?	This clever play on words for a dry-eye study involving eye drops focuses on the possibility of a solution for the condition vs. just symptom relief, and provides immediate recognition for the condition being studied.
Imagine Holding on Without the Pain of Rheumatoid Arthritis?	This message incorporates the condition being studied while combining symptom relief and the possibility of improved function, the primary motivator for this patient population.

There is also an art to getting the right media mix to promote the message. In addition to selecting the right radio stations and newspapers, advertisements have to appear at the right time and with the right frequency. And, when using other modalities, such as patient advocacy groups and health fairs, the recruitment handouts must be attractive, easily understandable and presented by the right person who can connect with the audience. These are factors that elude hardcore data analysis, yet are just as important to a successful recruitment campaign as finding the right sites. Think of the elegant restaurant that has wonderful food but poor service. Both are needed to create a positive experience.

New Ideas

The young patient recruitment industry is continually seeking new ideas to improve recruitment processes. In addition to the scientifically based early planning approach, there is a trend toward collaboration among outsourced partners, and an interest in developing patient recruitment forums to share ideas and increase professionalism within the industry.

The trend toward collaboration is a result of recruitment becoming more complex. As recruitment campaigns pull from various resources, there is a growing recognition that research organizations stand to benefit if multiple recruitment providers work together to optimize recruitment outcomes. This need to collaborate reflects the increasing specialization of providers, meaning that a single provider is generally not positioned to offer all of the required services, and must, therefore, reach out to other vendors. The pool of needed skills may represent an alliance among a recruitment provider that develops strategy, a healthcare information company, a media company to plan and make media buys, a web-based recruiter, a call center and a graphics design firm.

As a study unfolds, information from the various partners will flow to a central point, either to the contracted CRO, the sponsor or the recruitment provider. The CRO or sponsor may select all of the partners; or a recruitment provider may be chosen, and that company then moves forward with picking a call center, a web-based recruiter, a graphics designer and possibly a media company to refine media placement throughout the project.

Bill Gwinn, Director of Clinical Trial Solutions at Medstat, a healthcare information company, sees a definite movement toward collaboration and explains that the types of collaboration are a function of the size of the trial. "For smaller trials, or for earlier phase trials, sponsors seem to continue handling everything in house, but for large, multi-center phase III trials, sponsors are outsourcing functions more frequently to get the array of skills they need," Gwinn says.

Frank Kilpatrick, President of Healthcare Communications Group, a patient recruitment provider, considers the collaborative process as having two distinct levels. "There's the shotgun marriage, or the quick coming together of larger players, such as a CRO and a sponsor for a specific program. In this case, various partners may be assembled, such as a patient recruitment company, a web-based recruitment provider, or whatever is needed for a specific study. But real collaborations leading to genuine relationships from a strategic perspective are still very rare in this industry," Kilpatrick explains.

Real relationships between a sponsor and consultant revolve around a high level of data sharing and process sharing that is disclosed, usually confidentially, to achieve the desired results. According to Kilpatrick, obtaining clarity on issues such as an accurate data funnel, data sharing on site contribution, and information for creating an accurate budget can be hard to come by, but it is exactly this type of information that consultants need to

108

best serve their clients. "We are asked to solve a business problem—enrolling patients—and when we have accurate information, we can work together from a strategic perspective to make sure that recruitment happens on time. This makes everyone look like a winner, but most sponsors aren't there yet," says Kilpatrick.

Relationships that benefit the recruitment process may be formed from networking opportunities made available through new industry initiatives designed to increase professionalism in the field of patient recruitment. In 2003, the Drug Information Association (DIA) launched a Patient Recruitment Subcommittee within its Clinical Research Special Interest Area Community (SIAC). Co-chaired by Jim Kremidas of Eli Lilly & Co., and John Yee of BBK Healthcare, Inc., the subcommittee has a vision of being the leading forum for addressing the complexities of enrolling sufficient numbers of well-informed study volunteers into clinical trials on time and within budget. According to DIA, the subcommittee will focus on improving the operational skills of investigative site and sponsor personnel and increase industry awareness of the importance of considering enroll-ment, retention and compliance issues early and throughout the study design, planning and implementation processes.[13]

Kremidas says that this type of forum can serve as a central group or trade association for the industry, offering information about best practices in patient recruitment. The forum hopes to attract sponsor organizations, investigative sites, study participants and recruitment providers interested in improving how patient recruitment is conducted.

From the outset, the subcommittee defined its purpose (see Table 9) and its plans to measure its progress and impact. Kremidas comments, "A forum such as this might be of particular interest to sponsors, many of whom are changing the way they are approaching the question of patient recruitment. A number of sponsors are creating centralized recruitment groups, whereas in the past they didn't have this function in-house."

Table 9: Goals of the DIA Patient Recruitment Subcommittee

- Define metrics for measuring progress
- Use data-driven analysis to identify and share best practices among participants
- Develop and implement educational programs and communication tools
- Interface and provide input to other organizations regarding ethical issues associated with the enrollment of volunteers into clinical trials
- Develop and implement patient-focused communications regarding the risks and benefits of volunteering for clinical trials

Source: www.diahome.org

At the time of this writing (late 2003), the Association of Clinical Research Professionals (ACRP) is formulating and gearing up to launch a Patient Recruitment Forum. ACRP forums are designed to serve its members in specialty areas by providing professional interaction, ways to network effectively, and access to continuing education.[14]

According to Thomas Adams, CEO of ACRP, the goals of the patient recruitment forum have not yet been established, but a mission statement is in the development stage. "The forum will probably have its first meeting in conjunction with the annual meeting in May 2004. At that time, the group will determine how they want to operate, how frequently they want to meet, and what their direction will be," Adams says.

In addition to the DIA and ACRP initiatives, there is talk of a third patient recruitment group being formed, this being more of an independent trade association. Because it is in a preliminary stage, it is not clear if this association will get off the ground or if it will be truly independent or associated with a trade organization. If it does materialize, it has some specific intents. Gregg Sweet, of Integrated Clinical Trials Services, one of the individuals spearheading the effort, explains that this group might work toward bringing standards of excellence to the industry by encouraging development and adoption of standards of practice and standards for evaluating success. The organization might also provide an educational platform to the pharmaceutical industry, investigative sites and the general public.

Summary

Successful enrollment in the hypothetical osteoporosis trial, or for any trial, is the result of sites and sponsors seeing patient recruitment as a professional discipline, based on scientific and artistic principles. Science, which is about observing, measuring and interpreting phenomena, and art, defined as a system of principles and methods set up to perform a series of activities, are related practices, and may be thought as two sides of the same coin.

Although industry experts peg patient recruitment initiatives as having scientific and artistic components both, the orientation is scientific-leaning at this early stage in the industry's growth. Scientific methods are being used increasingly to pinpoint which recruitment techniques are most reliable and predictive of meeting enrollment targets. Metrics, for example, are being used to suggest the media mix to be used to achieve greatest impact for the dollar. As the study unfolds, media selection can be modified as necessary and analyzed after the study.

Informatics providers offer a range of scientific-based capabilities, such as testing the feasibility of a protocol for its recruitment potential by running the inclusion/exclusion criteria against massive databases to determine if enough patients exist to fill the study as designed. In addition, informatics providers can map the geographic prevalence of the disease in question and locate physicians and investigators in high prevalence areas with active practices and large numbers of patients in the therapeutic area of interest. Using these techniques, companies may be able to improve site selection, the key to a successful patient recruitment campaign, and to the clinical development program, overall.

Metrics and informatics databases are tools that reflect the growing use of evidence-based recruitment practice, mirroring the trend toward evidence-based medical practice. This strong scientific directive is laying the foundation for patient recruitment as a serious and professional discipline, however, that does not dismiss the important artistic, intuitive element that is needed to balance a dispassionate, all science approach.

Intuition is a critical factor, and so are an artistic eye and ear to craft the right message. Scientific evidence may point to the precise mix of media for the optimal recruitment campaign, but there is still the need to reach out and touch people in a way that stirs their interest in study participation. There is an art to doing this, to developing recruitment materials and advertisements that are visually appealing, have emotional pull to attract patients and pass regulatory scrutiny.

Some newer processes of patient recruitment illustrate the scientific and artistic basis of the discipline. Early planning is a technique, which, as the name suggests, highlights the value of starting the recruitment initiative very early, basically as soon as the sites are selected. Rather than waiting until sites are initiated to determine how recruitment will be done, the investigator meeting may be the ideal time to be proactive by soliciting investigator opinions for the best way to recruit. The science is in collecting, tallying and analyzing the information from the investigators. The art is in developing the messages and the appropriate materials. The process is in working with the sites to customize the approaches and in relationship building to encourage buy-in.

Relationship building is happening throughout the industry. As studies become more complex, providers need to collaborate to amass the full range of services required for success. The recruitment provider may work with an informatics company, a media company and a call center, for example. The networks created by these working relationships can be fostered as the industry moves toward the development of professional associations and forums. Industry groups are in the formative stages, but once up and running, they are deemed to establish guidelines for best recruitment practices, and standards for important industry trends such as collection of metrics and criteria for appropriate site selection.

Patient recruitment processes are changing. They are becoming more sophisticated, and more responsive to the demands of meeting global enrollment goals in a timely manner.

Key Takeaways

- Patient recruitment is a science and an art.
- At this point in the development of the patient recruitment industry, there seems to be more of an emphasis on scientific techniques, such as metrics and informatics, to improve site selection and investigator selection.
- The art of patient recruitment is most evident in the crafting of the right message.
- Early planning is a proactive, interactive exercise that seeks to meet enrollment targets on time and on budget by encouraging investigators to participate in the early structuring of recruitment campaigns that affect their sites.
- As clinical trials become more complex and recruitment providers become more specialized, there are likely to be more collaborations among them in order to supply the array of recruitment services needed.
- Patient recruitment forums are being organized and may provide members with opportunities to network and develop standards for best recruitment practices and metrics.

References

1. *The American Heritage Dictionary,* Second College Edition, Houghton Mifflin, 1982.
2. *The American Heritage Dictionary of the English Language,* Third Edition, Houghton Mifflin, 1996.
3. *The American Heritage Dictionary,* op.cit.
4. Ibid., *The American Heritage Dictionary.*
5. *The Brush and the Compass, The Interface Dynamics of Art and Science,* Paul Z. Hartal, University Press of America, 1988, p. 262.
6. CenterWatch surveys of investigative sites, 1997, and 2001.
7. American Medical Informatics Association, www.amia.org/about/faqs/f7.html, accessed October 7, 2003.
8. *Optimal Site Identification to Reach Patient Groups,* Beth Harper, Marcus Evans Conference, August 4, 2003.
9. *Implementing Proven Early Planning Recruitment Practices to Overcome Recruitment Challenges,* Diana Anderson, Ph.D., and Len Rosenberg, Ph.D., R.Ph., Barnett Conference, October 2003.
10. *President's Message, Balancing the Science and Art of Medicine,* Robert J. Lull, M.D., San Francisco Medicine, May 2002, Vol. 75, No. 5, www.sfms.org/sfm/sfm502k.htm, accessed October 7, 2003.

11. "Evidence-based medicine. A new approach to teaching the practice of medicine," Evidence-Based Medicine Working Group, *JAMA*, 1992; 268:2420-2425.
12. *Op.cit., President's Message, Balancing the Science and Art of Medicine.*
13. Drug Information Association, Clinical Research SIAC, www.diahome.org/doc/Communities/Community_sub_list_detail_T81 _R2/cfm, accessed October 9, 2003.
14. Association of Clinical Research Professionals, www.acrpnet.org/ network/forums/index.html, accessed October 10, 2003.

Author Biography

Diana L. Anderson, Ph.D.
President and CEO, D. L. Anderson International, Inc.
Dr. Diana L. Anderson is the President, CEO and Founder of D. L. Anderson International, Inc., parent company to subsidiaries D. Anderson & Company, a patient recruitment provider and RRI, a Contract Research Organization. D. Anderson & Company, the patient recruitment arm of D. L. Anderson International, Inc., provides a comprehensive menu of specialized services to the clinical trials industry. These services include consulting and patient recruitment management, market research and feasibility assessments, media management and purchasing, creative development, regulatory management, clinical trial branding, community outreach and public relations, site-specific recruitment services, direct-to-consumer strategies, call center support and retention programs.

Dr. Anderson consults globally as a recognized authority in the field of patient recruitment, with recent presentations in Japan, Europe and Israel. She is widely published and frequently featured for her accomplishments in a variety of trade publications and scientific journals. She is also the author of the books *50 Ways to Cope with Arthritis, A Guide to Patient Recruitment* and *A Guide to Patient Recruitment and Retention.*

Dr. Anderson serves on several corporate boards and in various capacities on committees including Immediate Past Chair of the Association of Clinical Research Professionals (ACRP). She has previously held appointments on the Board of Directors of the North Texas Chapter of the Arthritis Foundation; Editorial Board, *Arthritis Today Magazine*; Past President, Association of Rheumatology Health Professionals (ARHP); Board of Trustees of the National Arthritis Foundation; Board of Directors, American College of Rheumatology; and Past President, Western U.S.A. Pain Society. She maintains memberships and remains actively involved in a number of these professional organizations.

She holds a Ph.D. from Texas Woman's University, M.S.N. from the University of Texas Health Care Science Center in San Antonio, Texas, and a B.S.N. from the University of Nebraska.

C H A P T E R

Media Buying for Patient Recruitment

Evan Brett, Vice President, Clinical Trial Media

Objectives
- Discuss the effectiveness of patient recruitment media buying as it relates to expedited trial enrollment.
- Explore how patient recruitment advertisers can effectively use mass media.
- Identify the advantages and disadvantages that radio, broadcast television and newspaper advertising have to offer patient recruiters as an advertising medium.
- Examine the importance of negotiation, media management and response-driven creative execution as it relates to the effectiveness of a media purchase.

Introduction

Finding patients for clinical trials almost always begins with the examination of available patient databases and anticipated physician referrals. While in some cases, these resources are all that are needed to enroll a study, for the vast majority of studies they do not provide nearly enough subjects. For this reason, the effective use of mass media is routinely prescribed as the most productive method to recruit subjects. This chapter will explore how patient recruitment advertisers can effectively use mass media. Through a comprehensive discussion of media buying, discussion will identify the advantages and disadvantages that radio, broadcast television, and newspaper each has to offer as an advertising medium. The importance of negotiation, media management and response-driven creative execution as it relates to the effectiveness of a media purchase will be examined.

This chapter will focus on how effective patient recruitment media buying, that is, the process of researching, planning and purchasing advertising for clinical studies, can expedite trial enrollment.

Why Mass Media?

For purposes of discussion, the term "mass media" will be used to mean radio, broadcast television and newspaper outlets. These are usually the top three media vehicles used by patient recruitment advertisers because mass media, when purchased effectively, is a highly productive means to recruit potential subjects.

The success of mass media for patient recruitment can be attributed to three key factors.

1. Mass media permeates many aspects of everyone's lives. We rely on it for news, information and entertainment.
2. Mass media reaches a huge population. Because of the growing need for study subjects and increasingly difficult study design, massive numbers of potential subjects must be reached in order to reach recruitment goals.
3. Mass media provides an advertiser the ability to generate an immediate or "direct" response. This is a "call to action" where the advertisement generates a phone or web-based response to the message.

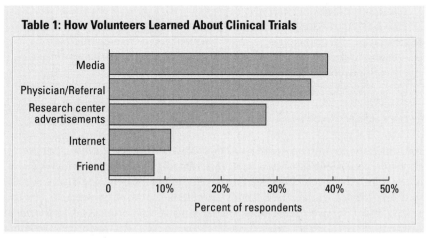

Table 1: How Volunteers Learned About Clinical Trials

Source: CenterWatch Survey of 1,565 Study Volunteers, 2002

For these reasons, sponsors, patient recruitment vendors, CROs, SMOs and sites routinely rely on mass media advertising to provide the requisite subjects to enroll their study. Centerwatch data indicate that 40% of all subjects learn of trials through the media (see Table 1).

Media Options

Television, radio and newspaper are the three key options to consider when using mass media to recruit subjects. The following section will cover the advantages and disadvantages of each medium, as well as provide counsel as to how and when to employ them properly.

Broadcast Television

Broadcast television's greatest attribute is that it reaches the largest audience of all three media. This is particularly valuable to clinical study advertisers who need to target a large population of individuals in order to obtain enough qualified participants.

Television also provides the advertiser an opportunity to reach their specific demographic by carefully selecting programming that will effectively reach the target audience. These factors may include age, gender, socioeconomic class and ethnicity. This is the key to using television to an advertiser's advantage. For example, a pediatric ADHD study targeting suburban, upscale, educated mothers ages 35-49 may be more appropriate advertising on *Dr. Phil*, *Oprah* and *The View* as opposed to programs such as *Jenny Jones* and *Jerry Springer,* which typically attract a younger, less sophisticated audience.

The programming time periods (dayparts) that have traditionally performed best for patient recruitment are early morning (7AM-9AM), daytime (9AM-4PM) and early news (4PM-6PM). Daytime is typically the least expensive daypart and offers a large variety of programs that allow the advertiser to choose appropriate programs for a target audience. Although daytime does not have the largest viewing audience of the day, it almost always generates the most cost-efficient response. It is important to note that daypart time periods vary by market and costs widely vary (see Table 2).

It is important in larger TV markets such as New York, Los Angeles and San Francisco to have multiple sites that are well dispersed within the metropolitan area in order for television to be used effectively. For example, it may be a mistake to use television in Los Angeles for only one site that is not centrally located. Remember, local television viewership spans a vast geographic radius and a subject will be more likely to participate and comply throughout a study if the travel distance is reasonable. Having multiple sites is not as important in smaller and midsize cities because travel time, traffic congestion and travel costs are not as significant in these areas.

Table 2: The Advantages and Disadvantages of Television

Advantages	Disadvantages
■ Sight, sound, color, motion	■ Waste due to broad demographic and geographic reach
■ Sense of immediacy, call to action	■ Advertising investment can be cost prohibitive
■ High reach medium	■ Cost of commercial production can be prohibitive
■ Ability to target specific demographic groups via specific station programming selections	■ Message has no shelf life

Radio

Radio has numerous attributes that can help explain why it is an excellent direct response medium for patient recruitment. Undoubtedly, it is part of most people's lifestyle. We wake up with radio and most rely on it for news, traffic, weather and entertainment in our home, car and workplace.

Radio Fact

Radio is typically sold in 60-second units, called spots.

Radio provides an opportunity to reach a specific demographic, psychographic and geographic target through format selection. For example, an adult 45-64 years old is likely to listen to News, Talk or Oldies formats, whereas an adult 18-34 often listens to music stations such as Top 40 music. News and Talk formats have historically been most effective at generating listener response. This is due to "foreground, active" listenership. People listen to News and Talk for spoken content, not music, so they need to pay close attention to what is being said. Talk formats consist of a large variety of programs hosted by local and national personalities. These options allow an advertiser to choose a topical program to reach their target audience. For example, a financial talk show that provides investment advice to seniors, or a news program, are appropriate advertising vehicles for such studies such as memory loss, geriatric depression, etc. Clinical study advertisers can also use radio to target listeners by ethnicity and geography. Wherever there is a concentration of an ethnic group such as Latinos or African Americans, it usually follows that an applicable radio format is available to serve the community.

Although the target audience of each study may have different listening habits, one fact remains the same. The most efficient subject response is generated during typical office hours (9AM-5PM), more specifically during the midday daypart, 10AM-3PM. Compared to drivetimes, midday listenership is lower, but the costs are relative. Although ratings are lower for midday, cost efficiency is greater. For this reason, middays should be the key component of a radio station purchase for direct response (see Table 3).

Table 3: The Advantages and Disadvantages of Radio

Advantages	Disadvantages
■ Effectively reaches listeners in transit to work, at work or at home	■ Can't see the message
	■ Not as broad reaching as television
■ Ability to isolate specific geographic region surrounding a site	■ Message has no shelf life
■ Sense of immediacy/call to action	
■ Target audience selectivity through Arbitron ratings and format analysis	
■ Opportunity to advertise in programming hosted by well-respected and credible show hosts	
■ Minimal production cost	

Newspaper

The use of local daily newspaper advertising as a direct response medium for patient recruitment is quite common because it offers a clinical study advertiser a variety of sections to reach the target demographic. These sections can include Main News, Health, Sports, Business and Entertainment, etc. There are also opportunities to run adjacent to specific content such as Advice, Horoscopes and Food.

Newspaper offers advertisers an opportunity to reach their target audience in a tangible format that enables a reader to "tear and clip" a patient recruitment advertisement for later use or to pass on to another person.

It is common to purchase a mix of weekday and Sunday advertising. Weekday advertising is less expensive than Sunday because the Sunday circulation of most newspapers is usually the largest of the week. It can make sense to buy both within a seven-day period because newspapers typically offer a "repeat discount" within the same week.

Print Fact

Print is sold by the column inch (ci). For example, if an advertiser runs a 2 column inch advertisement (one column commonly = 2 ⅛" and varies by publication) by 5", this would represent a 10 column inch ad (2ci x 5"=10"ci).

It is also wise to request outside positioning on the page so that the reader can easily tear out the ad if they are interested in calling at another time or passing on to someone else. They are less likely to go through the trouble if it involves making a mess of their paper.

Compared to television and radio, newspaper is less cost efficient. This is mostly due to newspaper's inability to generate as large a response as electronic media. Newspaper's cost is relatively high compared to the number of people it reaches. Despite this fact, it remains a staple of the patient recruitment community, more commonly, for sites. There are a few key reasons for this trend:

- Advertising budgets often leave no other choice. Many times an insertion or two in the local paper is all a site can afford.
- Newspaper is much easier for the layperson to buy than electronic media because it is priced according to a rate card and its pricing is more consistent.
- Sites often sign annual contracts with newspapers and need to fulfill commitments in order to avoid a year-end penalty, called a short rate.

With that said, newspaper can be a good choice in certain circumstances (see Table 4).

A common obstacle that clinical study advertisers face is the location of sites relative to the media market.

The following comments illustrate the previously described Los Angeles example discussed in the television section, where only one site was located in Los Angeles, and television was not advised. Hypothetically, if the site was in Orange County, 20 miles south of Los Angeles, the use of the *Orange County Register*, Orange County's local newspaper, is likely a better choice than buying television, or radio advertising to support this site. Although Orange County is technically a part of the Los Angeles market, it is unreasonable to expect that the majority of the Los Angeles population would travel to this distant site. Thus, *The Register* would be a more efficient and less expensive investment.

Table 4: The Advantages and Disadvantages of Print

Advantages	Disadvantages
■ Reader can "tear and clip" advertisement	■ Typically not cost efficient
■ Ability to target demographic audience via specific sections	■ Does not elicit an immediate response
■ Use of niche publications to target a reader (i.e., Senior News for Alzheimer's)	■ Poor return on investment
	■ Does not break through clutter
■ Ads can contain numerous details	■ Inability to capitalize on emotions
■ Reader can pass on to others	■ High cost relative to readership

Negotiation

Media is a negotiable commodity. The goal of a media seller is to obtain the highest price for his or her product, while the goal of a media buyer is to pay the least for it. The constant battle for a low price can be won with knowledge, clout and negotiating expertise. However, negotiation is not necessarily limited to pricing. No charge commercials/print insertions, advantageous cancellation rights, specific programming and ad positioning are all negotiable (see Table 5).

If a clinical trial advertiser tracks advertising response (which is highly recommended), it is important to communicate this to the media. Making the media accountable for response can motivate them to provide advantageous pricing and positioning. The station or publication is now aware that it must produce a cost-efficient response, or it risks a future cancellation. Since no media seller wants to lose revenue, the advertiser now has much greater leverage in a negotiation

Table 5: The Difference Between Electronic Media and Newspaper Pricing

Electronic media is more negotiable than newspaper. This is because newspaper is typically priced according to a rate card (pricing schedule) whereas television and radio pricing fluctuates daily, based on supply and demand. Newspaper, however, can always add a page to accommodate additional advertising and its pricing is not predicated on inventory availability.

Media Management

Media management refers to an ongoing advertising response analysis of a media buy. Based on response data, a media buy can be modified to help maximize response and minimize wasteful spending. Such modifications may entail the canceling of underperforming media and reallocating of funds to additional media outlets.

The process of media management entails quantifying call response relative to the advertising expenditure by individual station or publication. This measurement is referred to as the cost-per-call (CPC).

It is the norm that most patient recruitment advertisers fail to manage their media campaigns effectively. As a result they are unaware of which media are providing the greatest return on their investment. Needless to say, an unconscionable amount of money is being wasted every day by patient recruitment advertisers who are not vigilantly monitoring their media purchases.

Table 6: Sample Radio Copy (60 seconds)

Have you or someone you know been diagnosed with Multiple Sclerosis in the past three years?

There is no cure for MS, however a number of investigational drugs are being tested for the treatment of this disease.

A research study is currently being conducted in your area and is seeking adults who have been diagnosed with MS in the past three years, but have not yet received treatment.

All qualified participants will receive study medication, all study related treatment and follow up exams at no cost—and health insurance is not needed to participate. $500 compensation is being offered for your time and travel expenses.

So if you or someone you know has been diagnosed with Multiple Sclerosis call 1-800-MS-STUDY to learn if you qualify.

Remember, qualified participants will receive study medication, all study related treatment including MRI's and follow up exams at no cost—and health insurance is not needed to participate. $500 compensation is being offered for your time and travel expenses.

Call the toll free number now 1-800-MS-STUDY.

Once again, 1-800-MS-STUDY.

The Creative Message

While this chapter is focused on the media buying process as it relates to patient recruitment, this discussion would be incomplete without briefly touching on the importance of effective creative execution.

The following is a list of basic strategies to consider when creating a patient recruitment advertisement:

- Remember that the audience knows nothing about clinical research, therefore copy should be presented in layperson's terms.
- Straight copy, rather than humor or dialogue, break through the clutter and capture attention.
- Begin with common symptom questions if the study is targeting a naïve audience (e.g., Do you suffer from sleeplessness, fatigue and hopelessness?).
- Include what is being offered to the subject at no cost.
- Mention compensation or travel expenses if they are being offered.
- Mention that health insurance is not needed to participate.
- Mention that the call is toll free if applicable.
- Include site name to gain credibility if the study is being conducted at a prominent institution such as an academic hospital.
- Address family, friends and caregivers—"If you or someone you know...."

Table 7: Sample Television Storyboard

Anncr:	Have you or someone you know been diagnosed with Multiple Sclerosis in the past three years?
Super:	Diagnosed for the past three years
Anncr:	A research study is currently being conducted in your area and is seeking adults ages 30-45 who have been diagnosed with MS but have not received treatment.
Super:	Adults ages 30-45
Anncr:	All qualified participants will receive study medication, all study related treatment including MRI's and follow up exams at no cost and health insurance is not needed to participate. $500 compensation is being offered for your time and travel.
Super:	No cost to you
Anncr:	So if you or someone you know has been diagnosed with MS, call XYZ Research at 1-800-MS STUDY to speak with a research coordinator. 1-800-MS STUDY.

- Include emotions to touch the subject or loved one.
- When using radio, the phone number should be included three times and the message should end with the phone number.
- When using television, the phone number should be displayed throughout the commercial.
- When using print, the insertion should not be too small or too large. Ten to fourteen total column inches have proven to be effective without over- or underspending.

Table 8: Sample Print Ad

HAVE YOU BEEN DIAGNOSED WITH MULTIPLE SCLEROSIS?

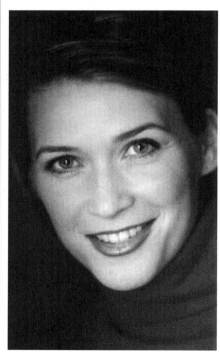

Have you been diagnosed with Multiple Sclerosis in the last 3 years?

If you have not received treatment, and are 30 to 45 years old, you may be eligible to participate in a research study evaluating the effectiveness of an investigational drug for the treatment for Multiple Sclerosis.

All qualified participants will receive study medication, all study related treatment and follow up exams at **no cost.**

Health insurance is **not needed** to participate.

Study participants will receive up to $500 for time and participation.

Call the toll free number now at:

1-800-MS-STUDY

XYZ
RESEARCH

XYZ Research, Inc. 5 Main St. Jericho, NY 07652

Summary

As the need for study subjects continues to grow, mass media will remain a necessary conduit for achieving drug approval. Mass media is not an inexpensive proposition and often represents the greatest cost of a recruitment campaign. That is why the success of a research study can be greatly influenced by the proper execution of a media purchase.

A thorough consideration of target demographic, site geography and advertising budget is needed to select appropriate media for a patient recruitment advertising campaign. The television programs, radio station formats and newspaper sections should be carefully selected in order to reach the greatest potential patient population.

It is important to negotiate the most attractive pricing and positioning in order to maximize an advertising budget. Once a buy has been executed, response data must be tracked carefully in order to modify media selections on an ongoing basis. This process will maintain media cost efficiency until the enrollment goal is met.

In conclusion, too many studies that suffer from recruitment inertia can benefit from an effective advertising initiative. This can mean the difference between a drug coming to market sooner, rather than later, which ultimately translates into a competitive advantage and increased revenue for the sponsor.

Key Takeaways

- The three key mass media options used to recruit subjects are television, radio and newspaper.
- There are advantages and disadvantages to television, radio and newspaper.
- Each has its own rationale as to how and when to employ them effectively.
- All media are negotiable and the objective of the buyer must be to purchase advertising with the best possible direct response exposure for the lowest cost.
- After a media purchase is implemented, an advertising campaign must be analyzed on an ongoing basis.
- An advertising campaign that follows all of the rules described in this chapter ultimately will not achieve success unless it is accompanied by a well-targeted, compelling and well-executed creative message.

Author Biography

Evan Brett
Vice President, Clinical Trial Media
Evan Brett is Vice President of Clinical Trial Media, Inc., a media buying company specializing in patient recruitment advertising. Evan co-founded Clinical Trial Media in 1995 to meet the growing need for media-based patient recruitment programs. CTM purchases media for pharmaceutical companies, patient recruitment firms, CROs, SMOs, research sites and advertising agencies. CTM has placed over $75,000,000 worth of media for patient recruitment campaigns covering a wide variety of therapeutic areas across North America. CTM has participated in the development of numerous compounds that have become some of the pharmaceutical industry's top performing brands.

Evan has presented on the topic of media buying at numerous patient recruitment conferences. He is a member of the Drug Information Association's Special Interest Area Committee on Patient Recruitment.

Evan graduated from the College of Public Programs at Arizona State University with a Bachelor of Arts in Broadcast Sales and Management. He has worked as a sales executive for KYOT-FM in Phoenix and for Blair Television.

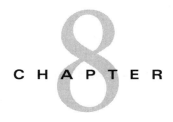

CHAPTER 8

Call Centers in Recruitment and Retention

Joseph Sameh, Founder of Phone Screen,
A division of American Mediconnect

Objectives
- Understand the difference between real-time and just-in-time data, and learn how to determine which is best for various communication tasks.
- Discuss how modern call centers implement converging technologies to improve the recruitment process and save sponsors recruitment dollars.
- Understand how call centers can be utilized beyond the screening process to support referral management and retention.
- Learn about how sites view centralized patient recruitment programs and their recommendations for improvements to the recruitment processes.

Introduction

Call centers long have been a key element in the patient-to-provider communications arena. The overarching goal of call centers is to save time (and/or money) for the provider while improving access for the patient. They are the originating source of a tremendous amount of clinical trials information. The value of this information increases with the accumulation of additional data.

Ultimately, call centers conduct the business of data acquisition and disbursement. They analyze performance metrics in a number of areas and serve the role of first contact point of data acquisition in the recruitment process. Call centers must work closely with all project partners, both upstream as well as downstream to realize the benefits available and thus add their value to the process.

Data Acquisition and Disbursement

Call centers foster rapid processing of data across multiple sites, markets, protocol, and media. They have also been called upon to help identify trends and implement solutions to recruitment and retention challenges. The term call center implies a phone call, but the phone call is no longer the sole source of data for call centers. Indeed call centers are often referred to and marketed as contact centers in their vastly transformed role as aggregators and disbursers of data. Institutional review board (IRB) review and approval are now required on all call guides. Further, HIPAA compliance statements along with existing standard procedures for the protection of patient and subject privacy should be available from call centers that are considering providing recruitment and retention services to the industry. (See Chapter 3 for more on the HIPAA Privacy Rule.)

Data attributed to and collected by call centers are generated at several points and by various methods. The acronym CTI once intended for computer telephony integration may be more appropriately defined today as computer, telephone and Internet connectivity. These three reference points indicate the various source points of data that converge at the call center.

The acquired data may be selectively categorized as system data, project data and meta data and further categorized as input/output devices. **System data** are data collected automatically by the Automatic Call Distribution (ACD) system or telephone switch. **Project data** consist of information acquired during the process of the call, or interaction with the call center. **Meta data** refer to the aggregate data and organizational analysis that occurs.

System Data
Many ACD systems passively collect more than fifty fields of data for each call within their system. The vast majority of this information plays little to no surface role in the overall process but certainly can inform and improve the process. The nature of these data includes information about the call itself, time and date of call, caller ID acquisition and duration of call. These are but a few of the data elements germane to the process. Much of the remaining information gathered passively is for the use of the call center and is most frequently utilized for diagnostic and quality control purposes.

Project Data
Project data are generally acquired during the screening by telephone agents (operators). These agents may have varying degrees of healthcare expertise depending on the nature of the study. Nurses or other healthcare specialists may be used when more complex healthcare questions are requuired during

the screening process. During a screening transaction, it is not uncommon to acquire more than one-hundred pieces of information per screen. Call centers aggregate data acquired by Interactive Voice Response Systems (IVRS), live telephone agents and the Internet.

Interactive Voice Response Systems (IVRS)

Interactive Voice Response Systems (IVRS) may be thought of as intelligent voice mail, or database driven voice mail. It combines all the possibilities of voice mail and integrates those with intelligent decision-based control. IVRS can reduce the demands on live screening substantially. Much information that is acquired during a phone screen can be captured effortlessly by IVRS. Examples include; gender, date of birth and zip code along with any information that may easily be acquired through a touch-tone phone. Ongoing subject surveys are a perfect use of IVR and can be orchestrated as either inbound or outbound calls.

Internet

The Internet screening component may be in the form of email, web chat, or web screening. Email submissions need to be screened completely as email offers no opportunity for a question/answer environment. Web chat presents the agent at a call center the opportunity to partially screen a candidate via an interactive process similar to instant messaging. Web screening provides the ability for a self-directed pre-screen prior to the call center's phone screen.

Live Screening

Live screening may be conducted in a stand-alone mode (no integration with other data sources) or integrated mode. Sophisticated call centers can aggregate information from the above sources into a single converged database as it occurs (real-time). Increasingly, studies may require a combination of efforts to achieve recruitment success. Today most screening tools are browser-based allowing sponsors to test-drive the call guide from their desktop prior to implementation. A sample screen shot of part of a call guide follows (see Table 1).

Meta Data

Meta data are analyzed retrospectively as a tool to foster improved accuracy in forecasting prospective recruitment rates. A call center with significant experience in a particular therapeutic area can assist the project partners with information to improve the likelihood of success.

Project planners can obtain accurate call duration estimates from prior similar study experience. Media planners can review anticipated call response rates based on prior media strategies. Media buyers can review previous response rates on a media outlet (station) basis. Service levels required by the protocol or sites may be identified at this point in time.

Table 1: Sample Live Screening Tool

> ### MEDICATIONS
>
> Are you currently taking any of the following medications?
>
> | | |
> |---|---|
> | ☐ Finasteride (Proscar, Propecia) | ☐ Dutasteride (Avodart) |
> | ☐ Anabolic Steroids | ☐ Spironolactone (Aldactone, Aldactazide) |
> | ☐ Flutamide (Eulexin) | ☐ Bicalutamide (Casodex) |
> | ☐ Cimetidine (Tagamet®) | ☐ Ketoconazole (Nizoral, topical ketoconazole is acceptable) |
> | ☐ None of these | ☐ Does not know |
>
> [FAQ] Comments: [_____] [Caller Terminated]
>
> [Next –>]

The data necessary to improve recruitment rates are often within reach if not already acquired by the call center. It is often more a question of looking at the data and asking: Is there a trend here? Is information available that, if acted upon, can improve the recruitment process? Where are the bottlenecks and shortcomings? Are there enough candidates in the pipeline to complete enrollment? Are we in danger of over enrollment?

While under-enrollment causes delays, over-enrollment can have its own costly effects. According to Jim Kremidas of Eli Lilly, costs of over-enrollment include the time cost between the time right-enrollment (the proper number of randomized subjects) and the study completion by the last randomized subject. Add to this the hard costs of additional grants to investigators, potential need of additional study materials (including drug compounds), and advertising costs associated with unnecessary study promotion and you can begin to reckon this cost. Early identification of potential enrollment problems (both over and under) can be better accomplished through centralized recruitment programs.

Reporting

When considerations of reporting and data delivery are taken into account, decisions must be made to determine best use and time requisite of data. Data are typically delivered by fax, email or through a secure, password-protected Internet application. Some applications demand real-time, dynamic oversight for best performance while other data needs require data at a specific point in time (just-in-time).

Real Time vs. Just in Time Data

An example of reasonable use of just-in-time data is the patient screen form sent to investigative sites. Candidates may pass the telephone or web screen outside of investigative site operating hours. The act of transferring referral forms to a site in real-time in the evening will not result in any benefit to the site, candidate or study. Indeed, forms transferred to the site immediately upon call completion (real-time) open the possibility for the site coordinator to overlook some referrals since each referral is faxed separately when delivered in real-time.

Sites commonly require screen pass information for processing during the next business day. Sites that can process screened candidates as the screening occurs may find an advantage to real-time delivery of phone screen information. Usually this is not the case. Therefore batch processing, or faxing all referrals for a predetermined period of time may be the best method to manage this segment of the recruitment process.

Many other decisions are best made by reviewing available data as it is presented. Without question, media buying decisions are best managed with data provided in real-time. As advertising runs in the media, the media buyer has the ability to compare and benchmark radio, TV and print media, outlet by outlet (station by station). Careful review and timely reallocation of underperforming media outlets can make a marked difference in the ability of a protocol to meet its recruitment objective.

Delivering Data

Project data are often delivered to project partners utilizing secure Internet connections. Data usually include all referred screened callers as well as those screen failures who have assented to be contacted for future studies. Data may be transferred in batch mode on a periodic basis (every day at midnight) or in real-time as each call is completed.

Screening—Processing the Call

Call processing begins when a call enters the Automatic Call Distribution (ACD). The main function however of the ACD is call routing. This routing capability is driven by account and agent properties. Account properties are managed by the phone number dialed and include routing parameters. Routing can direct a call to IVRS or a live agent. Routing alternatives can also be implemented by time of day to achieve greater efficiencies. An example is the routing of calls to a voice mail system when no screeners are on duty as in the middle of the night. Agent properties may be described as skills-based routing. Skills may include linguistic proficiency or gender preference based on study design.

When a call is transferred to an agent, a screen automatically appears that has been assigned to this protocol. This screen automatically provides the call guide (script) to the agent for screening.

When considering central recruitment, service levels must be defined. These service levels relate to expectations of call volume processing for the duration of the project. Service levels should be realistic and recognize the nuance of the protocol. Anticipated call volume must match the investigative sites ability to process referrals. Service levels may include time of day call processing, language spoken, gender and staffing levels.

Interactive Voice Response Systems (IVRS)

More advanced call centers have the ability to provide seamless transition from IVRS to a live agent while passing the IVRS-acquired data along to the agent. This integrated model provides significant financial benefit to the sponsor since IVRS time is considerably less expensive than live-agent time. Secondary advantages include the ability to process calls differently based on other parameters.

Intelligent Routing

One example of intelligent IVRS integration is the ability to rout a call differently if it is not the first time this caller has placed a call to this study line. The process includes development of a database of calling numbers (Caller ID). Each time a call enters the system, the system acquires the Caller ID and verifies that this is a first-time call from this number. The Caller ID is then added to a database since it is unique. Screening then proceeds normally.

In the event that the Caller ID already appears in this database, it is indicative that more than one call has originated from this source. Reasons for this may range from a previously disqualified caller attempting to alter some answers in an attempt to qualify for the study; a previously screened and referred candidate that has not been contacted by the investigative site; or multiple people using the same phone to screen for the study.

Unchecked, a repeat call from a previously disqualified person can affect the site with bad data. These people will clearly fail the screen at the investigative site. If excessive referrals persist, the time burden to everyone involved, from the call center to investigative site in processing can cause negative misperceptions of call center value to the recruitment process.

Referred candidates who have failed to receive a call or other communication from an investigative site frequently call the screening number a second time. These calls provide valuable insight about investigative sites' ability to process the number of referrals they are receiving from the call center.

Duplicate appearances of a phone number do not always indicate a problem. Pediatric studies are but one example of a study category where multiple screenings may legitimately originate from a single phone number.

Second calls may be automatically identified by the IVRS system immediately upon calling and routed automatically to site support or appropriate staff at the call center or site.

Web Screening

Generally speaking, there are two basic types of clinical trial web sites, active and passive. Passive sites provide information about studies and links for further information or listings of participating investigative sites. Passive sites may provide an email notification of interest or a web chat opportunity with a screener. Often these sites work with a call center to provide rapid response to the inquirer.

Active web sites provide a screening instrument that may look similar to a phone screen and ask similar questions. As a result, referrals may be similarly qualified. Joshua Schultz, co-founder and Vice President of Corporate Development of Veritas Medicine states "Having an online outreach and screening mechanism provides an incremental cohort who wants more information about a study prior to making a call. Therapeutic areas that preserve a social stigma are ideal for this type of recruitment."

Increasingly, web-based recruitment firms are partnering with call centers to aggregate data from multiple sources and provide for a standard method of delivering fulfillment materials to those candidates.

Live Screening—The Phone Screen

Live screening may involve screeners with varying degrees of medical expertise. Each protocol will determine the skill level required. Regardless of the level of medical expertise, a well-written and -ordered script will produce the best results for all involved.

A well-designed call guide will allow for the appropriate questions and answers that will not only deliver high probability (to randomize) referred patients, it must provide valuable data as well to, among other things, confirm the accuracy of the planned recruitment funnel.

A great irritant to screened callers is the lack of follow-through from the investigative site. These callers will tend to contact the call center a second time after passing the screen but failing to be contacted by the site. Second calls initiated by successfully screened candidates may be reduced or eliminated by offering a screening visit appointment at the time of phone screen. Appointments may be in person, via telephone, or in a group setting. When taken in aggregate, the seamless processing of multi access point interactions (web, IVRS, live) coupled with single-point management (screening, scheduling and confirmation) will translate to improvements in recruitment and retention efforts.

Predicting Enrollment

With knowledge of the data sets acquired during the screening process, the next logical question is, What can we do with the data? Predicting enrollment is the natural next step. It is both an art and a science. The costs that accrue due to late and under enrollment are well documented. Predicting enrollment is a task well suited to the delivery of call center data combined with site-based experience. An accurate model can assist the project team in controlling costs and time factors of a study and help identify study milestones earlier in the process.

In predicting enrollment there are several aspects to be considered.

- What percentage of advertising respondents (candidates) will pass the initial phone screen?
- Of those passing the phone screen, how many will pass secondary screening at the investigative site?
- What percentage will enroll and randomize?
- How many people are in the recruitment pipeline?
- Where in this process is each site and market?

Referral Management

Generally speaking, a call center's major role is to answer media postings of a protocol. The successfully screened candidates are forwarded to the participating sites. Occasionally, sites may be unable to process the referrals in a timely fashion. Frequently study candidates aren't available for phone calls during traditional office hours.

Referral management includes the act of communicating with screened study candidates to support investigative sites through the enrollment and randomization process. Call centers participate in referral management in various ways. One method of referral management is a weekly recapitulation of all referrals to each site with candidate status. Sites receive a summary, complete the form and fax it back to the call center. Other methods include Internet-based tracking of referred candidates. Typically, sites are expected to follow up with candidates within two or three days of passing the phone screening. In the event of unsuccessful attempts to contact, call centers will often provide referral management support in the form of a follow-up phone call to move the patient to the next level of recruitment (if appropriate).

Tables 2-4 specify a three-stage recruitment "funnel" indicating in succession the phone screen, site based secondary screening and finally screening visit to randomization phase. The funnel begins with the universe of potential candidates for a study and ends with enrolled and randomized subjects. Potential subjects drop out of the funnel for various reasons and at different steps along the screening and randomization continuum. The funnel really concludes with project closeout.Other than passive referral tracking, this study did not provide for active intervention.

Table 2: Funnel—Phone Screen

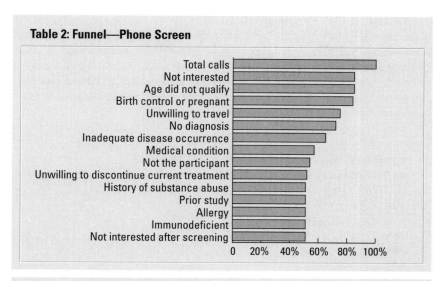

Table 3: Funnel—Secondary Screen

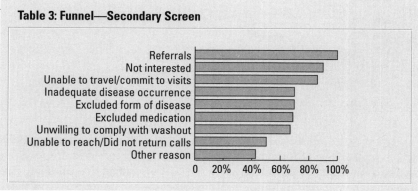

Table 4: Funnel—Screening Visits to Randomization

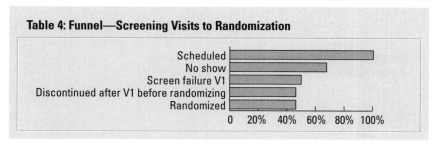

Tables 2-4 show the breakout of the overall recruitment funnel into three separate funnels representing the three screening points for this multisite, double-blind placebo-controlled study. Phone screen was conducted by a call center. A secondary screening was conducted via phone interview by each site. Successful patients were then scheduled for site visit. Each funnel begins with 100% of the people entering that phase.

We can see that 51% of callers passed the phone screen, 41% passed the secondary telephone screen and 46% of those scheduled for a site visit enrolled and randomized. Therefore, we can draw the conclusion that for every ten screened callers we will have one randomized subject (51%/41%/46%). For every five referred candidates we will have one randomized subject (41%/46%). For every two scheduled candidates we will have one randomized subject (46%).

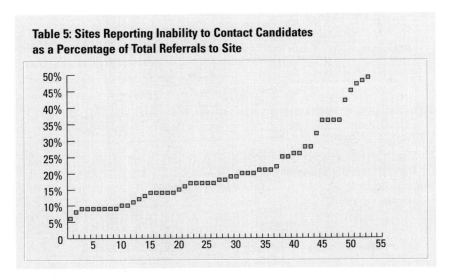

Table 5: Sites Reporting Inability to Contact Candidates as a Percentage of Total Referrals to Site

Upon closer examination it is noticeable that within the secondary phone screen phase, 18% of the candidates that did not proceed were dropped out due to an inability of the investigative site staff to contact the candidate (see Table 5). During the randomization phase we notice that fully 31% of those scheduled for a site visit failed to show up for the visit (see Table 6).

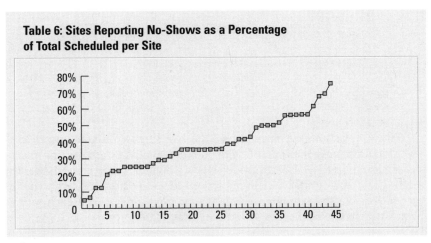

Table 6: Sites Reporting No-Shows as a Percentage of Total Scheduled per Site

Sites participating in this study have had a varying degree of difficulty contacting screened and referred callers. Sites reporting difficulty contacting these people ranged from 6% to 50% of all referrals per site. It should be noted that it is with a reasonable amount of certainty that for every five of these contacted there will likely result one randomized subject. Sponsors would do well to provide referral management support as an enhanced call center service to make every practical effort to maintain contact with the candidate. The relative importance of people in the funnel increases the further along the funnel we progress.

As we progress down the funnel, there are fewer people dropping out, and their value to study recruitment grows. In the third segment, sites reported appointment no-shows ranging from 5-71% of total candidates scheduled. By reviewing the randomization rate for this sub-group, we can determine that roughly 50% of patients entering this aspect of recruitment ultimately randomize into the study. Therefore, this group should be provided additional support in terms of communication including reminders and other support items that may spur participation.

In the event that enrollment and randomization are progressing according to the timeline, call center support for referral management may be minimal. In most cases, task assignment to a call center will improve the referral processing rate.

Working with Media

Media teams are responsible for creating and placing advertising that make the phones ring at the call center with likely candidates for a study. Their research informs message and media placement. Advertising source is one of the most important elements of non-clinical screening data captured within the call center. In order for the media buyers to do a good job, the call guide must provide for acquisition of rich information about media response. It is not enough to identify the source as radio, but rather, which radio station.

There are a number of methods that may be implemented to capture accurate media source data. Each media outlet may be assigned a unique advertising response telephone number. While beneficial to the automatic acquisition of data, this method is not always suitable in multi-market, multi-media studies where many phone numbers must be inventoried and managed.

A more common approach is to list one phone number for the study across all sites. Under this scenario, screeners must ascertain the type of medium (television, radio, newspaper, Internet, direct mail) by asking the caller. To be truly effective however, the media source (channel, newspaper, web site name, mail code) should be acquired as well.

Audiences don't always define their media choices in the same way. A radio station, for example, may be an affiliate of a major network referencing those call letters (ABC, CBS, NBC, etc.). This same radio station may have its own unique call letters (WLS, WGN, WNEW). In addition, each station has a position on a radio dial (102.7 FM). Finally, stations may be identified by their format (easy listening, talk radio, news radio). The same rules hold true for television. A well-designed script will include all station identifiers listed above to assist the caller in identifying the media source within their perception of the station.

The active management of media placement will produce better results than a program planned completely ahead of time.

Rate of Enrollment

Another role of media-call center interactions relates to particular investigative sites' ability to process referrals. During the active marketing of a recruitment campaign, a large number of referrals may be assigned to a site during a brief period. Sites may become overburdened by this sudden influx of candidates.

Repeat occurrences of second calls to the call center should be analyzed and reported to the project partners. If repeat callers indicate a delay at the site, media buyers should be made aware of the possibility that the site in question is receiving too many referrals, and advertising should be reviewed and perhaps adjusted.

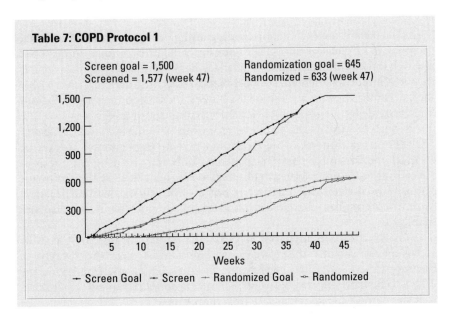

Table 7: COPD Protocol 1

Screen goal = 1,500
Screened = 1,577 (week 47)

Randomization goal = 645
Randomized = 633 (week 47)

Weeks

→ Screen Goal → Screen → Randomized Goal → Randomized

Table 8: COPD Protocol 2

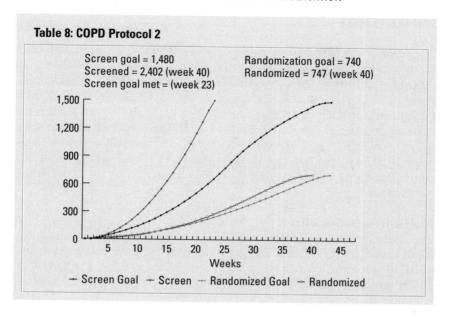

Screen goal = 1,480
Screened = 2,402 (week 40)
Screen goal met = (week 23)

Randomization goal = 740
Randomized = 747 (week 40)

— Screen Goal — Screen — Randomized Goal — Randomized

Tables 7 and 8 reflect two studies with identical compounds, and similar protocols, number of sites and number of subjects.

The recruitment goals of both studies were identical. The studies differed in approach and involvement of the call center. The first study used a call center for screening only. The second study added real-time online reporting, dynamic advertising management and close site communications. The accelerated rate of patient accrual is clearly evident. The second study closed advertising three months early at a savings of almost 30% of the total advertising budget. These studies underscore the major impact that high quality media and site relations can effect.

Disqualification Data

Precise identification of disqualification reasons can serve many purposes. A primary purpose is to test the hypothesis of the recruitment funnel. Disqualification data may pinpoint areas of concern. In the event that significant numbers of candidates opt out due to site distance factor, we may consider that the media net is too wide for the therapeutic area under study.

The vast majority of recruitment advertising is accurately targeted. Occasionally, disqualifications may be significantly out of sync with expectations indicating a misunderstanding of the advertising message or poorly written call guide. Protocol interpretation may play a role when subjective disease levels can contribute to varying rates of disqualification.

Retention

The major focus of attention within clinical trials in regard to the call center has been about recruitment. According to Richard Musselman of AvAMed Consulting Group Inc., "Study managers need not only budget for patient enrollment but they also need to budget for the things that keep patients enthused about staying in the study until the end. Clinical sites need to be made aware of the need to emphasize this to their potential study subjects at the beginning of the study. A strong and continual retention campaign in a long-term trial that includes newsletters, site training and other communications to study subjects will help to keep everyone engaged for the duration."

Fulfillment Services

The operative term in retention efforts is communication. This communication comes in many forms. The goal is to make the study subject look forward to continue participation in a long-term trial or a study with challenging compliance criteria.

Tools include:

- Newsletter delivery
- Appointment reminder calls to subjects
- Appointment confirmation calls to subjects
- Appointment reminder mail/email to subjects
- Appointment confirmation mail/email to subjects
- Study hot lines (live and web based) for subjects
- After-hours investigator access
- Real-time adverse event reporting
- Appointment-window reminders to site or subject
- Inbound and outbound quality-of-life surveys
- Exception reports to CRO/sponsor
- Educational materials
- 24/7 appointment scheduling
- Combine elements of patient education to terms of study compliance
- Referrals to advocacy groups

Key Takeaways

- Call centers are a key element in patient-to-provider communication.
- Call centers acquire and disburse clinical trials data as well as analyze performance metrics.
- Predicting enrollment is a task well-suited to the delivery of call center data combined with site-based experience.

- A call center's major role is to answer media postings of a protocol; referral management includes the act of communicating with screened study candidates to support investigative sites through the enrollment and randomization process.
- Advertising source is one of the most important elements of non-clinical screening data within the call center.

Author Biography

Joseph Sameh
Founder of Phone Screen, a Division of American Mediconnect

Joe Sameh is a serial entrepreneur with more than 30 years of experience in computer, telephone and communications systems, primarily in the health-care environment. A recognized industry leader, author and frequent speaker at professional conferences, he is a specialist in applying technical solutions to human interface and process improvement methods.

Nationally, authorship includes peer-reviewed articles in call center and drug development publications, as well as contributing author for the industry handbook, *A Guide To Patient Recruitment* (Centerwatch, 2001). Sameh has been mentioned in *The Chicago Sun Times*, *Wall Street Journal*, *PharmaVoice*, *The Monitor*, and *CWWeekly* among others. He has authored articles in many call center publications including *Connections Magazine* and featured in *Teleconnect Magazine*.

Accomplishments include the development of the centralized recruitment concept (Phone Screen—1991—www.phonescreen.com) for enhanced performance accelerated subject recruitment for clinical drug trials. Another innovation, On Line Reporting was the first Privacy Rule compliant real-time reporting tool in the industry (1999).

Experience in presentation includes Illinois Teleservices Association, Great Lakes Teleservices Association, Drug Information Association, Rush Pres. St. Lukes Medical Center, Johns Hopkins, Association for Clinical Research Professionals, University of Illinois Center for Enterprise Development and National Amtelco Equipment Owners, among others. Sameh has experience as an expert witness relating to healthcare call center issues.

Other involvements include local and regional civic leadership, including weekly visits to a nursing home and participation in programs to feed the hungry.

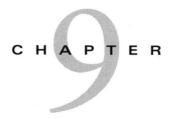

Budgeting and Contracting in Patient Recruitment

Bonnie A. Brescia, Founding Principal, BBK Healthcare, Inc.

Objectives

- Budgeting and contracting that incorporates patient realities during the earliest stages is essential to the success of clinical trials.
- Developing distinct strategies and understanding budget variables and components leads to effective patient recruitment budgets.
- Understanding and identifying a company's values are key parts of the budget process.

Introduction

In the field of patient recruitment for clinical trials, considerations of budgeting and contracting are becoming increasingly essential to success. This chapter challenges clinicians, administrators, sponsors and others involved in clinical trials to think more strategically in deciding when, where, how and why to budget and contract for patient recruitment.

Until recently, patient recruitment was exclusive to the principal investigator's role in a clinical trial. Patients for clinical trials were largely drawn from the physician's practice, and the sponsor paid for that access as part of the physician's total compensation. A separate budget for centralized patient recruitment was rare.

As the number of clinical trials increased and competition grew among companies testing similar compounds and procedures, recruiting patients from physician practices was not enough. It became necessary to find new methods for attracting participants. Individual study sites began spending money on promotional campaigns with widely varying degrees of success. For every success there were more failures, and the duplication among sites of effort was inefficient and wasteful.

Management within sponsor organizations soon began analyzing the return on investment for patient recruitment efforts, challenging the marketplace to re-evaluate the concept of decentralized versus centralized campaigns and budgets. The first organizations to attempt centralized programs were contract research organizations (CROs). However, CROs lacked expertise in direct-to-consumer promotions, and soon it was necessary to find others that could analyze the process and develop a marketing communications strategy for patient recruitment as a distinct effort. Many early, centralized recruitment budgets were often inflated, even exorbitant. More recently, the pooling of patient recruitment expertise distributed throughout the clinical trial community—sponsors, sites, CROs, site management organizations (SMOs) and communications agencies—has resulted in a more strategic approach to budgeting for patient recruitment.

This need for achieving recruitment success in an efficient, cost-effective and process-oriented manner has led to the growth of strategic contracting as a budget management tool. Performance-based contracting among sponsors, sites, CROs and communications specialists is an effective method for distributing the risks and rewards—without unduly influencing the informed consent process involved in the increasingly competitive field of clinical trial recruitment.

Every protocol demands its own budgeting strategy. What follows is a process to assist project leaders in understanding the variables that affect the recruitment budget, which, when evaluated, lead to a comprehensive patient recruitment budget.

Before Budgeting

In one successful study after another, a commitment to investing in patient recruitment at the onset has achieved demonstrable results: expenses can be anticipated, allocated and contained. Furthermore, patient involvement and retention in these studies have increased. Rather than planning protocol design, investigator recruitment or patient recruitment as sequential steps in a process over time, when all elements are considered early and concurrently, a study can be more effectively managed. Ultimately, this mindset shift from linear to dynamic planning has proven effective in avoiding the recurring problem of under-enrolled studies. This section provides an overview of key questions to ask about the trial, specifically:

- Is there a method for estimating numbers of patients needed at each recruitment stage to fulfill the final randomized requirement?

- What are the factors essential to determining budget size and scope?
- Is the decision to use a centralized or decentralized budget?
- What are the options of competitive recruitment for sites?

A review of these issues will pave the way to drafting a strategically sound budget.

Answering Key Questions

Before creating a patient recruitment budget, it is necessary to develop a protocol recruitment profile by answering several key questions. Keep this profile as a reference throughout the recruitment planning, budgeting and contracting process. Answer these questions now and refer to them while reading the next few sections.

1. How many randomized participants are needed?
2. How many patients must be screened to enroll the target number?
3. How many sites are planned?
4. Where will the sites be located geographically?
5. How much of the recruitment effort—if any—can the sites handle?
6. Is this study pivotal (e.g., providing data for NDA?) or is it an earlier phase?
7. How important is the product/compound to the company's business strategy?
8. Does the company have recent recruitment experience in this therapeutic category?
9 What is the time frame for beginning and completing the study?
10. How onerous are the inclusion/exclusion criteria?
11. What is the incidence of the disease/condition?
12. Are there competitive treatments currently available?
13. Are all sites under a central IRB or individual IRBs?

Determining a Recruitment Funnel

In order to recruit the target number of enrolled patients for a study, a much greater number of potential participants must be reached through promotional efforts. This larger pool of candidates will be evaluated based on their eligibility and appropriateness for the study, creating a "funnel" effect. Before developing a patient recruitment budget, it is important to make assumptions about the recruitment funnel for each study. These assumptions provide initial performance metrics against which a program can be measured. They also form the basis for many decisions that will affect program design and allocation of resources. Essentially, this model projects the number of individuals who must respond to a promotional program in order to generate a target number of patients who will pass through the various screens and ultimately be randomized into a study.

The first step in using the recruitment funnel method is to determine how many individuals an investigator is likely to see for a medical evaluation in order to enroll (randomize) one patient into the study. These funnels are rudimentary feasibility analyses. They are a first look at the practicability of the protocol and the achievability of the study recruitment objectives. However, for a true recruitment feasibility analysis, more complex modeling is required to reduce the probability of error in the funnel.

Understanding how many people must be reached to effectively enroll the target number of patients has a significant effect on the budget. The protocol promotional profile is an analysis of the ways in which the protocol design actively assists or inhibits the potential for patient recruitment. A thorough understanding of the key points that may appeal to or repel patients, allows a projection of the numbers required within a recruitment funnel. For example, in a diabetic neuropathy study, ten patients might need to be screened in order to enroll one patient. However, the promotional campaign may need to reach 1,000 people in order to generate the ten qualified callers that will result in one enrolled patient. In this scenario, the ratio of callers to enrollees may be so great that the investigative site may be understaffed to generate or respond to this volume of inquiries. Thus, the budget would be expanded to allow for additional personnel or the use of a centralized response center to field patient inquiries.

Table 1: The Recruitment Funnel

Stage of Enrollment	Numbers needed to enroll/randomize one individual	Numbers extrapolated to enroll/randomize 750 individuals
Inquiries	24	21,000
Referred to sites	8	7,000
Made and kept appointments	6	4,500
Medically eligible	2	1,500
Enrolled/Randomized	1	750

It should be noted that not every individual referred to a site for medical evaluation will make and keep an appointment. Next comes the determination of how many people must pass a preliminary screening for key demographic and basic medical history in order to be appropriate for an in-person medical evaluation. Last is the determination of how many people are needed to call the study site or central toll-free number in order to generate the desired number of individuals who will pass the preliminary screening. See Table 1 for an example of how the recruitment funnel works.

Use of the recruitment funnel can also serve as an early feasibility assessment of employing marketing communications tactics to achieve recruitment goals. If it becomes apparent from this type of analysis that a significant percentage of the potential patient pool (i.e., more than 5%) must respond to marketing communications, then it may be necessary to consider more significant strategic recommendations in addition. For example, other strategic tactics could include reducing the number of patients, broadening the scope of recruitable patients or increasing the number of study sites.

The complexity of the model is a reflection of the many variables that contribute to recruitment outcomes. These might also include:

- Length of the recruitment period
- Potential patient universe based on investigative site location
- Average number of investigative sites actively recruiting throughout the recruitment period
- Patient panel sizes of principal investigators
- Average number of incident cases at each investigative site
- Competing studies at investigative sites
- Probable patient outreach response based on budget
- Inclusion/exclusion criteria
- Willingness of the principal investigator to recommend the study as a treatment option
- Percentage of eligible patients that will go on to participate in the study

This list is far from exhaustive. It does not include the effect of the study coordinator on recruitment (which may or may not be significant based on the type of patient outreach deemed necessary to satisfy the recruitment parameters of the study). Furthermore, enrollment may be dependent on additional factors, including the therapeutic category, sponsors, investigative sites, CROs, patient recruitment vendors and other external forces.

Considering Budget Factors

Evaluating the factors in a budget helps determine its size and scope. No matter the size of a trial, certain factors don't change. In any study, a certain level of strategy, research and development costs are required. Other factors are variable and depend on the number and location of markets, number of sites and patients and more.

Timing

The timing of when a budget is developed affects which elements can be included or must be eliminated because the timelines for their implementation fall outside the recruitment window. The earlier in the clinical trial process that the patient recruitment budget is considered, the more likely it is that recruitment will be accomplished in a timely and cost-effective manner. There are several stages when a patient recruitment budget is typically considered.

At Protocol Development

The earliest moment to consider the budget is concurrently with development of the trial protocol. Decisions about patient definition and selection, investment of time and other factors affect recruitment efforts. For example, rather than planning a trial with 100 sites in 100 different media markets, consider grouping the 100 sites in 20 media markets. Not only will this save in marketing costs, but in other expenditures as well. For example, travel costs for investigator meetings and site monitoring also may be reduced. Planning the budget at this point provides the most control over options and choices.

At Study Launch

This is a second common point at which budgets are developed. When patient recruitment is problematic at this stage, some options may be reduced. For example, sites are likely to be already contracted; thus changes in number and location of sites or modifications to the protocol to improve patient-friendliness may be too cumbersome to implement. But there is still an opportunity to bring a proposal to management and perhaps prevent some of the lost time and revenue that occurs in rescue mode.

Rescue Mode

Once the study has started and patient recruitment is recognized as a problem, the costs in time and effort for a supplemental recruitment program are at a premium. Advertising costs may be locked in at an expensive time of year. Some outreach options such as public relations may be unavailable because, although they are effective and cost-efficient, they require long lead times to implement and bear results. Marketing may be limited to less-than-optimum materials already developed and approved by IRBs, or new materials may need to be developed and approved dependent on the constraints of the IRBs. When options are limited, costs go up.

Difficulty of Protocol

Once the protocol is written, it can be used to estimate the recruitment cost per patient. There are factors in each protocol that make it easier or harder to recruit patients. Protocol factors that often increase recruitment difficulty include a placebo arm, satisfactory existing treatments in the therapeutic category being studied, one or more invasive procedures, and limited prevalence/incidence of the disease and resultant difficulty of subject identification. Factors that might make recruitment easier include likelihood of medical insurance coverage, no satisfactory existing treatments in the category, wide demographic population being studied, long lead time to study start date, and use of a central IRB.

Number of Patients/Number of Sites

Both of these factors increase costs incrementally. The more patients that are needed, the more money is required to recruit. Likewise, the more sites in the study, the more resources that must be allocated to cover the media markets and the costs of creating and producing materials. Each site has startup costs and each requires monitoring. Decisions must be made about whether to distribute promotion across more sites or limit the number of sites and provide more funds for promotion.

Location of Sites

Deciding on the location of sites will affect the budget. Locating multiple sites in one media market is a cost-saving strategy. Placing them in densely populated areas is another strategy to increase the number of potential participants reached with fewer dollars. Analyzing past and potential site performance is important to determine which sites would be most effective to include. Does the site have a dedicated recruitment specialist or marketing manager? If so, it's more likely they will know how to use promotional funds effectively.

Management Priorities

How important is the drug being studied to the Sponsor's overall business strategy? The answer will affect budgeting decisions. If the drug already has a revenue stream and the study will help to extend or expand that revenue stream, management will probably be more willing to spend money on recruitment to shorten the overall length of study duration. The same may hold true for promising new compounds with the first-to-market position at stake. Project leaders should not assume that because patient recruitment has not been budgeted as a separate effort in the past, that management would not support a sizeable recruitment budget today.

Choosing a Centralized or Decentralized Budget Model

One of the first considerations in setting a patient recruitment budget is to determine whether to use a decentralized or centralized budget, or a combination of both. In the days when sponsors contracted solely with physicians, recruitment budgets were managed by investigators and associated site staff. Under this decentralized model, clinicians managed the entire process of patient interaction, from initial recruitment, through the course of the study to collecting, analyzing and reporting data. Patient recruitment components, such as patient screening, special events and advertising, were line items in the investigator's budget. Pharmaceutical companies chose investigators based on their reputations, ability to recruit patients and proposed budgets. Over time, clinical trials became more competitive. Sites had to become more sophisticated and reach outside their own practices to recruit patients. Their costs went up and duplication of efforts became common as each site created its own versions of study and promotional materials.

Budget centralization was introduced to address these issues. In this model, the sponsor originated strategy and media materials and then communicated the message and disseminated the materials to investigators and sites. For direct-to-consumer campaigns, call centers were added into the budget to centralize patient screening and processing because the volume of respondents became too high for individuals at the sites to cope with.

Once the rule, decentralized budgets may soon become the exception. However, there are some instances that may make decentralization the optimum choice. When the number of participants in a trial is small, distributing recruitment funds to individual sites may be more efficient. If the study needs 85 patients from seven sites, providing each site with a budget of $10,000 to execute local promotion would still be less expensive than engaging a communications firm to develop a single campaign. It is reasonable to assume that sites will be able to deliver some percentage of the target number of patients from their existing practice or databases. And this higher-than-average allocation of promotional funds is likely to fill in the gap.

Allocating funds on a per site basis is also advantageous when a local effort is the most effective way to reach potential patients, e.g., a screening event, or when leveraging existing relationships is essential, e.g., using physician referrals to find patients. Decentralized budgets—which leave promotional responsibilities with the study sites—can also reduce the workload for sponsor staff as compared to centralized budgets, which sponsor staff must manage.

Centralizing the budget is often the most effective model for patient recruitment. Particularly for large trials and phase IIb or later trials, the benefits of centralization are many. Centralization offers economies of scale, requiring the performance of work only once and preventing duplication of efforts. Centralization also results in more effective tracking. When call centers are used to collect information as a central source, sponsors are not dependent on numerous sites to submit reports relating to recruitment promotional data. Project managers can determine early on whether sufficient resources are being deployed to generate sufficient number of potential study participants to meet enrollment. A weekly analysis of recruitment performance enables course corrections to reallocate budgets to the most effective strategies or sites.

Management over the budget also gives sponsors greater control over promotional content. When investigators supervise the budget, there may not be a mechanism for sponsor review and approval of promotional materials. In an era when regulatory energies are being focused on investigator ethics in recruitment, sponsor-initiated, IRB-approved campaigns may provide greater control over regulatory compliance.

Sometimes, a combination of centralized and decentralized budgeting works well. For example, a trial might be launched through a centralized TV or radio campaign and then followed up with sites running print ads as needed to complete enrollment. The choice of centralized, decentralized or combination budgeting for recruitment is a strategic decision that will affect the study's outcome as measured in time to completion and total cost to completion. This decision also will affect the contracts executed with out-source suppliers.

Deciding to Recruit Competitively or Not

Deciding how to motivate sites to recruit also affects the patient recruitment budget. With competitive recruitment, sites are rewarded financially for the number of patients they enroll. Media support is equalized across markets to provide a level playing field. Sites compete to recruit the most patients. An alternative approach is to budget fixed amounts unevenly among the sites depending on expected recruitment performance. In this model, higher performing sites are supported with higher budget amounts, ensuring higher recruitment rates. In both approaches, the funds to both support the promotional effort and reward the sites are allocated in the marketing and media portion of the budget. The promotional budget in either case may be the same, but there is a difference in how it is spent.

Knowledge of site performance is key when making the decision to choose a competitive recruitment or alternative model. If there is no history of site performance, then competitive recruitment might be a good choice. In competitive recruitment, the first sites to enroll the most patients are rewarded. Should there be knowledge and experience of various sites as proven high performers, allocating funds by known performance levels may make more sense. In this case, it is not as important to enroll patients first as to enroll patients at a consistently higher rate than other sites.

In the competitive recruitment approach, sites are challenged to recruit a minimum number of patients at a certain fee per patient evaluated, with the opportunity to increase earnings for recruitment over the quota. For example, if 500 patients are needed from 50 sites, Sponsors budget and contract for ten patients per site, but offer compensation for up to 30 patients recruited. Thus, the sites that are skilled at recruiting generate more revenue from their research effort. Less effective sites receive less or may be removed from the study. However, there are operating costs to administer a study even for a non-performing site. Spending more promotional dollars on fewer sites may result in a lower overall study budget. Again, the decisions made about recruitment have the potential to affect many line items in the study's operational budget that are not directly related to recruitment.

Table 2: Comparison of Media Costs, Target Market Women 25–54

Market (Rank)	Total Gross TV Costs/ 50 TRPs*	Total Gross Radio Costs 50 TRPs*	Sunday Newspaper Gross Cost, 3 col x 7"	Total by Market
New York (#1)	$37,388	$33,020	$19,887.56	$90,295
Los Angeles (#2)	$28,563	$41,950	$20,937.00	$91,450
Seattle (#12)	$9,538	$12,800	$7,468.23	$29,806
Birmingham (#40)	$2,863	$3,750	$3,401.79	$10,014
Tulsa (#60)	$3,050	$1,948	$2,709.00	$7,707

*TRPs=target rating points

TV daypart mix:
25% Early Morning, 25% Daytime, 25% Early News, 25% Late News

Radio daypart mix:
25% AM Drive, 35% Midday, 25% PM Drive, 15% Weekend

Broadcast Source:
2003 Media Market Guide (Spring issue); W25-54

Newspaper Sunday open rates:
SRDS May 2003

**New York Daily News*, a tabloid newspaper, is based on a 4c x 7" (28")

With this model, sponsors must be careful to provide equal promotional support to all sites. Support should be equalized by effort, not dollars. This means that sites in more expensive media markets may receive more money to reach the same target audience that a less expensive market may need fewer funds to find. While it may seem obvious that radio advertising in New York City is more expensive than in Tulsa, Okla., few decentralized recruitment budgets account for these wide variations in media costs market to market. Equalizing these costs across markets is done by assigning a target rating point or number of impressions for promotion in each market. Rating points represent the percentage of the marketplace that is exposed to an advertising message. Impressions are the number of people who are exposed to the message. Rather than budgeting a flat amount per site or per market, it is wise to consider budgeting for a number of impressions generated or percentage of the marketplace to be reached. See Table 2 below for an example of equalized support across different media markets.

In the alternative model, no effort is made to support sites equally. In fact, more promotional funds to support recruitment efforts are allocated to the sites that are already known to be the best recruiters. Based on site performance levels, sites can be divided into several tiers. At the lowest tier are the sites that may or may not reach their quota. They receive a set amount of promotional support. For sites that, with the addition of extra funds, can reach beyond their recruitment quota, more is budgeted. Top performers receive the greatest budget support. The extra effort ensures that the best performers recruit the most patients. Many project managers set initial budgets for the first ten patients enrolled. If a site demonstrates strength in recruitment, the project manager can use money from a contingency fund to further support that site in recruiting additional participants. This approach can be deployed within a centralized or decentralized budgeting model.

As in many other budgeting decisions, the approach to allocating promotional dollars by site (or market) can affect the overall outcome of other aspects of the study. Many project managers have found that competitive recruitment creates tensions within the clinical trial community despite efforts to equalize resources. And despite the initial inequities in the tiered support model, participating sites in these programs appreciate that some effort has been made to match study promotions with their capacity to manage the results of an outreach campaign.

Drafting a Budget

Having made pre-budgeting decisions, the process of drafting a budget is easier and more efficient. Using the knowledge gained, it is time to draft a budget. Although most organizations crave a budget standard for recruitment, there is no industry-wide accepted practice for patient recruitment budgeting. In the field, wide variations in budget allocations are seen.

At BBK, budgeting is approached from one of two perspectives. In one approach, the budget is built from the ground up depending on the assessment of the protocol and its recruitment challenges. In the other approach, a fixed budget is provided that is then allocated to provide the greatest return on investment (ROI).

In a "from-the-ground-up" budget, each protocol is evaluated to determine its relative difficulty of enrollment. Usually, this involves projecting the level of enrollment expected to be provided through site-based tactics (e.g., brochures, posters, patient database mining), which in turn indicates the enrollment gap (if any) to be filled through outreach tactics (e.g., advertising, direct mail, publicity, Internet). Subsequent analysis of patient populations suggests the kinds of outreach most effective, and how much such outreach will be necessary to "fill the funnel." Budgeting follows by costing the various components.

Often, managers have a fixed amount of money that can be invested in patient recruitment, regardless of evidence that might suggest a bigger budget may be necessary to complete enrollment. In this instance, it is important to evaluate all of the potential program elements on a return-on-investment basis. If it is determined that a single promotional activity has the potential to generate the most inquiries or randomize the most patients, then it may be prudent to allocate all of a $200,000 budget to a single promotional activity. However, a multi-tactical campaign is more complicated and the integrated communications within those campaigns tend to support one another rather than working separately. In a campaign with print advertising and direct mail, each tactic is likely to get a better response than would advertising or direct mail alone. Further, it is not unusual for a limited fixed budget to eliminate the tactic predicted most effective due to that tactic's high cost. For example: radio advertising may be projected as most effective per dollar, but since radio is a medium where effective results are determined based on frequent on-air messages, the investment necessary to produce, distribute and air a message may exceed the entire fixed budget. Fixed budgeting involves determining optimal allocations between the various recruitment campaign components judged most effective, given the overall limit.

When a direct-to-consumer promotional campaign is required to meet enrollment goals, an average of $1,500 per enrolled (randomized) patient is applied as a baseline for budgeting. For example, if 600 individuals must be recruited to an influenza study that has been assessed as having an average difficulty, $900,000 would be calculated as a planning measure. For a study that requires multiple endoscopies and has extensive exclusion criteria, it might be determined that the protocol has twice the difficulty of the influenza study. In this case, the planning budget would be based on an assumption of $3,000 per enrolled (randomized) patient.

Depending on the study, such cost per patient figures can be more misleading than helpful. Reasons include the significantly more competitive recruitment environment, as well as the increasingly esoteric protocol requirements. "Average difficulty" is far more difficult than it once was, and as a result costs per patient enrolled of $5,000 or more are increasingly common. Administrators, reasonably enough, are prone to balk at such figures. This is all the incentive many managers need to produce a careful but realistic analysis of recruitment needs. Often enough, even the higher recruitment costs pale in comparison to the operating costs or more certainly the lost opportunity costs of a prolonged enrollment period.

Some clients prefer to budget for recruitment using standards that have been set for other direct response advertising programs they have conducted. In these cases, the number of inquiries required is the critical factor in setting the budget. Target costs per inquiry can range from $50 to $250 (or more) depending on the percent of people in the marketplace who are eligible to respond to promotion based on having the condition under investigation. In this scenario, if 10,000 individuals are needed to call the toll-free phone number and the population is relatively easy to target, such as type 2 diabetics, then the budget might be set at $75 per inquiry, or $750,000 for the program as a whole.

Budget Components

This section outlines the common components of a patient recruitment budget and provides a budget worksheet that can be used as a planning tool when drafting a project budget. Depending on the size of the budget, not all components come into play, but all should be considered. Each component is followed by a list of representative expenses contained within it.

Research, Strategy and Planning: Focus groups, database searches, purchase of existing reports on therapeutic category and sufferers, consulting services (such as for protocol design) and population tracking and demographics.

Creative Development: Creation of a graphic identity system or study logo, preparation of materials including letterhead, brochures, print and broadcast advertisements, direct mailers, posters, flyers, web sites, etc. (Hint: Budget for creative development separately from production. Send all materials for regulatory and IRB approval at one time. Incur production costs on a phased, or as-needed, basis. Save money by not producing all materials until their deployment is warranted. Save time by not returning for supplemental regulatory/IRB approval in mid-stream.)

Production: Production of approved pieces from creative development; includes printing, copying and collating, production of radio or television commercials, talent fees, photography and/or illustration rights, web programming, etc.

Marketing and Media:
Media Placement: Ad space in newspapers, on the Web or in outdoor media; ad time on the radio, TV or cable; list rental; postage for direct mail programs, etc.

Publicity: Development of press kits, press releases and public service announcements. Separate charges will be incurred for distributing materials via mail or wire services. Professional fees for conducting media follow-up, coordinating news coverage and coaching study spokespersons.

Community Outreach: Participation in existing gatherings and events (e.g., health fairs, senior center meetings, church groups, etc.).

Internet Outreach: Creation of a web site with general study information and an online screener/referral application; purchase of keywords, listings and advertisements on major search engines; postings on electronic bulletin boards and newsgroups, listing and links on related sites, etc.

Special Events: Organization of study-specific events coordinated by the sponsor or sites.

IRB Approvals: Costs for approval differ depending on the IRB. Some IRBs will charge per item, some per campaign and others will negotiate volume discounts for review of the same materials on behalf of a multitude of sites.

Campaign Management, Project Management and Reporting: Coordination of campaign components, communication between managers, vendor, administrators, clinical teams, technology licenses for project management software, etc.

Metrics and Evaluation: Determination of measurable objectives, development of systems to track them, analysis of results, ongoing recommendations for redeployment of resources.

Call Center Operations: (Hint: Separate the fixed from the variable costs in the budget. In the fixed line item, include start-up costs and minimum monthly charges. In the variable budget, put all items that are tied to number and disposition of calls.)

Fixed Costs: Start-up fees, operator training, computer programming of screener, database design, standard report package, etc.

Variable Costs: Inbound operator costs (most often charged on a per-minute basis which will vary depending on the complexity of screening and level of personnel required), outbound calls, customized reporting, distribution and fulfillment of requests for information, customized services to support sites with patient scheduling, follow-up, appointment reminders, etc.

Site Support Services: Personnel liaison with sites, site training, hiring or subcontracting staff, coaching, newsletters, web sites, teleconferencing, patient scheduling, mailing, on-site staff, software, web-based applications for communication between sites, sponsors, referral tracking, IRB tracking, etc.

Site Incentives: Recognition gifts as allowed by sponsor or site management, thank-yous, newsletters, plaques, etc.

Patient Incentives: Compensation, parking stipends, books, gift certificates, newsletters, cards and communications, etc.

Miscellaneous Expenses: Out-of-pocket expenses, shipping and delivery, travel costs, teleconferencing, supplies, overhead charges, etc.

Other Budgetary Considerations

Hiring a Call Center

When a Call Center Is Mandatory
When a patient recruitment media campaign includes broadcast advertising and public relations, there is a potential to generate a large number of calls (fifty or more) per day. If it is a national campaign or covers more than ten media markets, this level of calls could persist for several days or weeks at a time. On their own, study sites would be unable to handle the volume. Calls would back up, potential patients would not receive callbacks and patients would be lost. To ensure candidates are responded to immediately and processed efficiently, a call center is essential. When spending $1 million on a media campaign to inspire callers, it is worth another $270,000 to ensure those callers are processed efficiently; otherwise, the effort could be wasted.

Choosing a Dedicated or Shared Environment
Professional call centers can be contracted to be dedicated only to one client or to answer calls for many clients. It is of course more costly to contract a dedicated call center, and it is rarely justified unless a company has multiple (over a dozen) studies in recruitment phase at the same time. Far more common are shared environment call centers, where operators take calls for many clients and studies. This way costs are shared; and there is no charge for down time when operators are not answering calls for a particular study.

Patient Recruitment Budget Worksheet
The worksheet below includes examples of budgets for comprehensive and moderate recruitment programs. Referring to the sections above, use the columns on the right side of the worksheet to draft a new budget or to organize a current program budget (see Table 3).

Table 3: Patient Recruitment Budget Worksheet

Budget Component	Outreach Budget %	Outreach Budget $
Research, strategy and planning	6%	$90,000
Creative development	4%	$60,000
Materials production	8%	$120,000
Marketing and media (media placement, publicity, community outreach, Internet outreach, special events)	43%	$650,000
IRB approvals	2%	$30,000
Campaign management	6%	$90,000
Metrics and evaluation	5%	$70,000
Call center operations	8%	$120,000
Site support services	9%	$140,000
Site incentives	2%	$30,000
Patient incentives	5%	$70,000
Miscellaneous expenses	2%	$30,000
Total		$1,500,000

After Budgeting

There are several considerations that follow the drafting of a budget. There will always be changes and unexpected circumstances that should be allowed for in a contingency budget. Many studies require ongoing maintenance in the form of efforts to retain patients, which may necessitate additional funding outside of the recruitment budget. In addition, once all of these budgets are complete, it is essential to gain the confidence and approval of management to go forward. The following section explores these areas.

Planning a Contingency Budget
No matter how thorough the initial planning, inevitably there will be changes during the course of the recruitment period that cannot be anticipated. Contingency budgets provide project managers with the resources to respond to changing conditions. However, not all organizations view con-

Site-Based Tactics Budget		Sample Budget	
%	$	%	$
11%	$40,000		
10%	$35,000		
11%	$40,000		
0%	–		
3%	$10,000		
9%	$30,000		
6%	$20,000		
0%	–		
40%	$140,000		
9%	$30,000		
0%	–		
1%	$5,000		
	$350,000		

tingency budgets in the same way. Some see planning a contingency budget as part of the process. Others perceive it as a sign of incompetence. Still others prefer to budget more money than is necessary in the main budget and then plan to spend only two-thirds of it. When planning the budget, it is important to know the nature of the organization involved. Generally, a contingency budget should be planned below the line of the main budget. Factors that require contingency might include the following:

Miscalculations: Not enough candidates are calling in, more are needed; or the target number of patients is calling, but qualification rates are lower than expected.

Not all IRB Materials Approved on Schedule: Approval may have to be sought in phases, with a percentage of sites receiving approval up front and the rest later. In this case, the recruitment efforts will be executed piecemeal, resulting in higher labor and production charges. Another effect of delayed approval could be delayed media placement. Since advertising rates change seasonally, a delay in project execution that moves a media placement buy from February to April could result in as much as a 20% increase in costs as second and third quarter rates are more expensive than first quarter. Fourth quarter rates are the most expensive of all.

Sites Added or Withdrawn: Adding sites increases costs in many areas, including patient recruitment; withdrawing sites may mean shifting budget amounts and burden to remaining sites; delays in sites getting protocol approval results in less time to review.

Changes in Protocol: These changes often affect the messaging, media and outreach efforts, e.g., if the age is changed from 18-70 to 12-70, the strategy must be adapted to reach a younger audience.

Considering Retention Costs

If a trial runs 26 weeks or longer, it is worth considering a budget for retaining patients in the study. For multiyear trials, a retention budget is mandatory. This should be a budget separate from patient recruitment and contingency recruitment costs.

To keep patients involved and motivated, it is important to budget for ongoing communication with them, as well as for investigators and site coordinators. It is helpful to solicit feedback from participants to determine the nature of communications or support they value most. Usually, they want more information about the study and how to best manage their disease state. Educational information makes participants feel valued. Carrying the study's logo or graphic identity on to the development of retention materials is a logical means of continuing the connection between study, participants and site staff.

Consider the call center a resource for retention as well, investing in training for follow-up calls, continued appointment scheduling and confirmation, surveys and polls. The call center can be a key tool in maintaining positive contact with patients.

As for patient recruitment estimating, there are no accepted industry standards for budgeting for patient retention. At BBK, costs per patient are estimated at $100 (US) per patient per retention year as a starting point in the planning stage. If the study is particularly complicated and requires more frequent interaction with patients, then a higher budget may be necessary.

Selling the Budget to Management

Even the most carefully thought out budget does not guarantee management support for new approaches to recruitment. It is necessary to understand the politics and dynamics of the management style of the organization granting approval. Knowledge of the company's previous experience, confidence level and commitment to a product or study is important in planning the strategy for achieving approval of the budget.

Outsourcing Supervisors: There is a growing trend in the pharmaceutical industry to identify internal individuals and departments as responsible for serving as resources and sometimes gatekeepers in the budgeting process. Based in the clinical, financial or communications areas of a company, they provide knowledge of outsourced resources, evaluation of outside suppliers, guidance through the competitive bidding process, negotiation procedures and more. Teaming with these experts and gaining their endorsement can be of great assistance in selling the budget to management.

One-Shot vs. Phased Approvals: Depending on the nature of the company, there are different strategies for seeking approval. If confidence in a budget is high, and the management has had positive experiences in budgeting patient recruitment, then one-shot, or comprehensive, budget approval may be possible. When confidence is lower, and the company may have had little or unsatisfactory experience with centralized patient recruitment, a phased approach might be best. Suggesting a $300,000 demonstration project on a $1.5 million budget could encourage gradual buy-in. Successful completion can be presented as proof-of-concept and full approval requested. Once again, it is important to understand the politics and preferred management style of the company.

Performance Projections: It is an easy and worthwhile exercise to anticipate management challenges to a patient recruitment budget. For each program element in a patient recruitment campaign, project the performance of that effort, calculate related costs and prepare performance metrics. These projections estimate the success of the recruitment effort. Examples include number of inquiries, referral ratios and number of enrollees. These numbers can help add meaning and convince management of the value of various media efforts, etc. Tables 4 and 5 give examples of performance projections by program and anticipated return-on-investment figures. While it may be easy to see that one method of outreach is far more cost efficient than

Table 4: Performance Projections

Source	Inquiries	Refer Ratio	Referrals to Sites	Enrolled
Site support	N/A	N/A	1,200	725
Publicity	1,000	4:1	250	75
Internet	2,000	8:1	250	50
Direct mail	500	3:1	167	50
Advertising	3,000	5:1	600	100
Total	**6,500**		**2,467**	**1,000**

Table 5: Return on Investment

Source	Budget	Inquiries
Site support and incentives	$240,000	N/A
Publicity	$200,000	1,000
Internet	$110,000	2,000
Direct mail	$120,000	500
Advertising	$340,000	3,000
Subtotal	**$1,010,000**	**6,500**
Call center	$120,000	4,500
Research, strategy and planning	$90,000	6,500
Creative development	$60,000	6,500
IRB approvals	$30,000	6,500
Campaign management	$90,000	6,500
Metrics and evaluation	$70,000	6,500
Miscellaneous	$30,000	6,500
Total	**$1,500,000**	**6,500**

another, rarely will that one method reach a sufficient number of individuals to achieve the total program goal. Typically, the first 50% of patients enrolled will cost less than 50% of the total promotional budget. Often, the final 20 percent of enrollees may require up to 50 percent of the total recruitment budget to identify and recruit.

Contracting

In the competitive environment of current patient recruitment practices, contracting is becoming an increasingly popular and essential budget management tool. Agencies work synergistically to achieve a common goal through strategic use of contracts, sponsors, investigators, sites and communications. Contracting can ensure the most effective placement and use of funds and provide a dynamic environment for executing budgets.

Contracts That Work
The most successful contracts include several factors.

Cost/Inquiry	Referrals	Cost/Referral	Enrolled	Cost/Enrolled
N/A	1,200	$256	725	$331
$200	250	$240	75	$2,667
$55	250	$240	50	$2,200
$240	167	$318	50	$2,400
$113	600	$455	100	$3,400
$155	**2,467**	**$409**	**1,000**	**$1,010**
$27	N/A	N/A	225	$533
$14	N/A	N/A	1,000	$90
$9	N/A	N/A	1,000	$60
$5	N/A	N/A	1,000	$30
$14	N/A	N/A	1,000	$90
$11	N/A	N/A	1,000	$70
$5	N/A	N/A	1,000	$30
$231	**2,467**	**$608**	**1,000**	**$1,500**

Scope of Service

Establishing a clear expectation of activities that are tied to recruitment is essential. It is not enough to simply hold sites responsible for recruitment goals. In the decentralized budget model, what portion should be contracted? Will sponsors pay sites for each patient they screen or only for patients enrolled? What if a site has to handle 200 calls to enroll 20 patients? In this case, payment per enrolled patient is a disincentive to achieve the volume of inquiries needed to complete recruitment.

Process for Change

Change is inevitable in the clinical trial process. Recruitment does not always follow the plan laid out, management makes changes, sites are added or dropped, etc. The most successful contracts build in a process for handling these changes. With a process in place, money can be added if patients are added, or shifted from print advertising to radio based on new knowledge of the target audience. The process for change should include a mechanism for proposal, justification, review and approval and should identify parties responsible for all steps.

Ownership

Contracts must cover the question of who owns the work. Most companies want to own the materials produced for a recruitment campaign. But "perfecting" complete ownership of work can be extremely expensive. The copyrights for a stock illustration or photograph could easily be $40,000. Licensing the use of the same artwork for a distinct period of time might be a fraction of the cost. The same is true of software, fonts and other elements. Advertising is not typically covered as work for hire. However, the agency or artist producing the advertising can be asked to assign the copyright to another entity.

Risk-Reward Contracting

Risk-reward contracts are tools for sharing the financial risk of recruitment for clinical trials and for managing budget concerns. As the stakes increase, risk-sharing agreements tied to a variety of objective and subjective goals are becoming more commonplace. Five basic models of risk-sharing contracts are described here.

Withholding

This model involves the buyer withholding certain payments until the supplier meets set objectives. That may include recruiting a set number of eligible patients into a clinical trial or increasing the sales of a particular drug by a preset amount. A withhold contract represents a risk-only approach that ensures the company does not pay until the supplier meets objectives. There is little incentive to suppliers—beyond gaining a new client—to accept such a contract, as it offers no reward other than payment for services if they meet objectives.

Bonuses

This model is the inverse of the withhold contract and is a more widely accepted risk-sharing agreement. It is a rewards-only approach that provides incentives to the supplier to meet or exceed expectations. That approach could include tangible expectations, such as recruitment of a specified number of patients into a program by key milestones set at the start of the program. Less tangible measurements could also serve as measures for bonuses, such as overall product awareness or even the working relationship established between the supplier and project manager.

Volume Discounting

The principle behind this model is that the vendor is guaranteed a certain volume of business and, in turn, the purchaser receives a lower per-unit cost. In other words, by committing to a guaranteed amount of business, the purchaser is able to take advantage of a lower cost and avoid spending the additional money required to find and establish relationships with multiple vendors. The supplier has a tangible commitment and is able to spend less time and money winning the business and more time servicing it.

Utilization Management

This model evolved from volume discounting. The guiding principle behind most risk and reward agreements is the notion of controlling utilization and increasing efficiencies. So that both parties undertake some element of risk and reward, utilization management is based on the principle of controlling overall costs to the client while providing increased unit pricing to the vendor. In those instances, the vendor is responsible for process control and education and for finding new and inventive ways for improving procedures and efficiencies to drive down overall costs.

Capitation

Examples of the capitation model include a cost-per-inquiry on a direct response program, cost-per-marketshare point gained or cost-per-sales increase. A cost-per-patient arrangement is ideal for clinical trial suppliers, as the trial sponsor can easily measure patient enrollment.

Elements of these various risk-sharing models can be deployed in patient recruitment contracting among sponsors and CROs, SMOs, individual investigators, communications agencies and call centers. The most successful risk-sharing arrangements are built on existing relationships where trust, clear communications and shared business goals are in place.

Summary

Creating a patient recruitment budget and considering contracting options are becoming ever more essential in the highly competitive and rapidly growing field of clinical trials. To successfully plan and execute patient recruitment budgets and contracts, there are several essential considerations. Creating a study profile and projecting a recruitment funnel from the framework on which a budget is built. Recognizing the importance of timing in creating a budget cannot be overemphasized in its effect on the scope and size of expenditures. When actually drafting the budget, all elements must be considered and the possibility of future changes incorporated into a contingency budget. Selling the budget to management is a critical step, the success of which often can be influenced by preparation and presentation of performance metrics, both before and after budget approval. To support and strengthen budget initiatives, strategic contracting is vital for reinforcing recruitment performance. By following a thoughtful, strategically sound budget plan into the clinical trial effort, recruitment becomes an increasingly integral part of the process and is much more likely to contribute to the drive toward successful drug and device development and marketing.

Key Takeaways

- Accelerating and improving patient recruitment for clinical trials at the earliest stages enables Sponsors to better anticipate, allocate and manage budgetary expenses.
- Early planning avoids the bottlenecks that hamper sponsors' ability to bring new products to market due to a critical lack of patient enrollment.
- Utilizing the recruitment funnel concept before finalizing a patient recruitment budget provides initial performance metrics against which a program can be measured.
- Prioritizing a patient recruitment budget around strategic, research and development considerations are crucial components of successful budgets.
- Considering a centralized or decentralized budget model, deciding whether to recruit competitively and balancing media placements ensure that costs are equalized.
- Keeping one's hand on the pulse of the budget after it has been completed is necessary in order to determine whether additional funding outside the recruitment budget is needed.

Author Biography

Bonnie A. Brescia
Founding Principal, BBK Healthcare, Inc.
As founding principal of BBK Healthcare, Bonnie A. Brescia has led the company's evolution as a marketing consulting firm for the clinical research and development segment of the pharmaceutical, biotechnology and medical device industries, helping to accelerate time to market for new medicines and treatments. A well-recognized thought leader in patient recruitment, she has firmly established BBK as a pioneer in developing marketing solutions that ease bottlenecks in the clinical development process.

With 25 years of marketing communications and financial management experience, Ms. Brescia ensures sound foundations for successful client campaigns. Under her leadership, BBK has earned a reputation for combining marketing science with research science to create clinical studies that enroll on time and on budget. Under her direction, BBK has also pioneered many advances such as TrialCentralNet[SM], an e-business application that optimizes management of patient recruitment campaigns. The firm's most recent initiative, Good Recruitment Practice[SM], establishes principles and best practices for Investigator and patient recruitment. Ms. Brescia also guides BBK's client development and relationship management efforts, offering consultation and direction in project development and implementation.

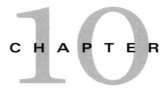

The Importance of Retention

John Needham

Objectives
- Discuss the importance and timing of conducting protocol feasibility research with potential Investigators and participants.
- Detail the challenges subjects may face while remaining enrolled and compliant, providing possible solutions to the challenges.
- Provide data points for a Recruitment Lessons Learned Database.
- Review the components of Recruitment and Compliance Kits.

Introduction

The successful implementation, management and completion of multi-center, global clinical trials depend, in large part, on the timely recruitment of highly compliant and protocol-adhering participants. It is prudent to ensure an edge is given to your study over those of other companies with competing products. That competitive edge could be the level of care and steady flow of educational materials that study participants, their family or caregivers will receive during the course of the study.

When recruiting participants, we sometime lose sight of the endpoint of our efforts: that we only submit *evaluable patient data* to our government regulatory authorities. So it is important to have a plan and a process for not only recruiting and enrolling the required number of subjects, but also ensuring that they follow the protocol regimen, take the medication when they are supposed to and as directed, and that they keep all their office visits.

The Participant Adherence and Retention Plan

The Participant Adherence and Retention Plan has to come from a review of historical data from similar studies and from market research focused on the patients most likely to meet the study criteria. In addition, sites should develop a process to identify and screen those potential participants at high risk for non-adherence and study dropout. Sponsors often neglect this phase of the study because they wait too long to plan a combined recruitment and retention strategy or inadequately fund it. Little effort is focused on how the site can keep participants motivated and address their needs throughout the study.

Retention plans are not just for studies that continue over a long period of time. Many studies require frequent site visits or each appointment may last for several hours, placing a burden on the participant, or caregiver. Retention programs are needed for studies with difficult dosing regimens, data collection, invasive procedures, extensive caregiver requirements and unpleasant side effects of the compound. Adherence programs supplement the retention programs by offering guidance on the proper dosing of the medication, the value of staying in the study and the importance of each site visit.

To improve the success of our trial efforts, we must understand many aspects of the participants' lives, medical beliefs, daily habits, moral convictions, disease seasonality and impact of the family on the potential participants. Adherence and retention will have barriers associated with them and they should be addressed.

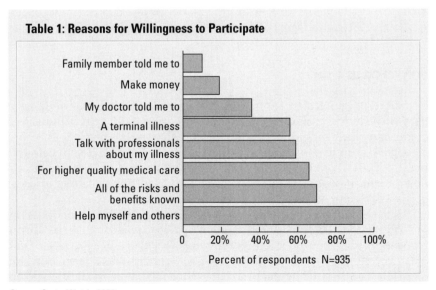

Table 1: Reasons for Willingness to Participate

Percent of respondents N=935

Source: CenterWatch, 2002

Patients join studies to improve their own health as well as to contribute to the advances of science and medicine (see Table 1). It is important to the potential participant that we provide a "study mission" communication early in the enrollment process to reinforce a participant's commitment to the trial's purpose. For the sponsor, protocol feasibility *must* be conducted before the protocol is finalized. Much can be learned from historical data (past performance of the principal investigator, enrollment per site per month, patient attrition), but each study is unique and little should be taken for granted. The team working on the compound may be new to this disease or it may be a patient population never studied before.

What affects adherence in clinical trials is not unique to the trial's environment:

- Patients take doses at intervals different from those prescribed
- Patients take "drug holidays," may over-medicate or dump meds before an appointment
- Side effects influence compliance
- Success is related strongly to how the dosing regimen integrates with their daily activities
- Adherence is not dependent on income levels, social class, occupation or formal education

Often, the critical elements of adherence are not addressed by the sponsor during the planning phase of the study or the feasibility assessment of a potential investigative site. The site's staff and investigators often don't anticipate the challenges their patients will face with this compound and therefore do not have a formal strategy to emphasize the importance of adherence and retention in the study.

The successful sponsor gathers market research data regarding retention and adherence from patients, former study participants, study coordinators, site monitors and investigators for every study.

Specifically:

- How long do people generally live with this disease and how does the disease affect their quality of life?
- Would a patient's personal physician recommend that they participate?
- What would the challenges be to full participation?
- How far would they be willing to travel to a site; what effect would winter weather have on their ability to complete participation?
- How long would they be able to participate: weeks, months, years?
- What duration would the ideal study visit be?
- What effect would a placebo arm have on their willingness to go off a current medication to join the trial?
- What would help them take their medication as prescribed—a reminder phone call or email, a watch with an alarm, a beeping pill bottle?

- Where should the sponsor focus its energies toward retention and compliance, and what materials should be offered the sites and the patients/caregivers?
- Does this patient population have altruistic views about clinical trials and if so, what message will motivate them?

This is a new approach, and a sponsor should look at these data to determine if the current protocol design will work and if the site will be motivated to offer an unprecedented level of care to the participants. If the answer is no, then the site-selection criteria needs to change in order to facilitate the enrollment and retention of the right individuals for this trial.

The best way for a site to prepare for a future study is to maintain a "Lessons Learned" database for each completed study, and segment the data by disease state. The sponsors should only select sites that can demonstrate that they thoroughly understand their patients by knowing how this disease affects their life and by changing their practice to accommodate the patients.

Responses to the following questions should go into the Lessons Learned database:

- How long has it taken in the past to complete enrollment?
- Where is the best place to find the participants?
- How many patients do I have to speak to in order to set one appointment?
- What are the most preferred days and times for appointments?
- What has been the average screen failure rate?
- How many people fail to show up for their appointment?
- How far are people willing to drive for their appointment?
- How many people drop out for non-medical reasons?
- What was the average length of their participation?
- How many people want literature and pamphlets before deciding to enroll?
- How many people have participated in more than one study?
- What methods were used to attract those patients?
- Have other physicians been willing to refer patients?
- Who generally makes the decision about participation—the patient or a family member?

Answers to these questions, accumulated over time, will build a strategy on how to approach the new study and provide the sponsor more accurate information in the feasibility questionnaire.

Adherence: Issues and Solutions

Patient motivation and behavior are too complex to be given one explanation or solved with one simple brochure. Because not one size fits all, several intervention strategies should be considered and combined to find the right mix of influences for each participant (see Table 2). Tailored communication support driven by the patient's needs lead to a better patient experience and hopefully improved study results.

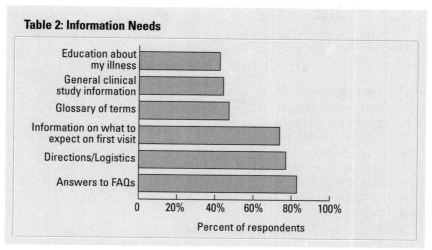

Table 2: Information Needs

Source: CenterWatch, 2002

During pre-screening, sites should focus on setting expectations at the outset of a patient's participation. Proactive sites provide potential participants with disease- or study-specific educational materials (Pre-Enrollment Kit) before they visit the site. They schedule only the pre-qualified, motivated patients. This helps eliminate the early dropout factor experienced when patients aren't properly advised of study requirements during the initial education and consent process. Sites should adjust their office hours to accommodate the busy schedule of the potential participant.

Cues to non-adherence often surface during the informed consent process. One solution is to assign a trained "pre-screener" designed to pick up cues to non-adherence and only select potential participants who are motivated and have the ability to adhere to the study design throughout the study.

Once a participant has agreed to participate and signed the informed consent, they should receive a "Welcome" Kit and immediately be made to feel that they are part of an important effort in which their contribution really counts (Table 3).

Once dosing has begun for the participant, it is important that sites make it clear that knowing what is required and doing it are two different things. Correct trial participation between office visits is a matter of "self-management." Both the investigator and the sponsor are totally dependent on patients' behavior and adherence to the study design to know if the compound is effective.

Table 3: Retention and Adherence Kits Components

Pre-screening Kit
- Directions to the site
- What to expect on the first visit
- Frequently Asked Questions (FAQs)
- Disease-/disorder-specific information
- Site contact information

"Welcome" Enrollment Kit
- "Participating in a Clinical Trial" brochure
- Specific trial information
- FAQs about the specific trial
- Comment card
- Expense reimbursement form
- Point of contact business card at the site
- Refrigerator magnet
- Patient personal organizer folder
- Patient contact information sheet for the site

Adherence/Retention Tools
- Holiday/Birthday card
- Appreciation gift (< $10.00)
- Milestone gift (< $25.00)
- Feedback/Evaluation cards
- Newsletter
- Patient follow-up letter from PI
- Appointment card
- Visit reminder postcard
- Missed appointment postcard
- Calendar with appointment stickers

Completion Kit
- Certificate of Completion
- List of resources (support groups)
- Thank you letter from PI
- Opt-in card for future trials

Web home pages for the disease

Sites should engage in ongoing discussions with the participants both during and between office visits on the challenges of the study. Every participant is different and each one should be offered educational materials in a way that fits their style of learning: aural or visual. Providing these materials in the participant's native language can contribute to a greater understanding of the information.

Participant Appreciation and Reinforcement Reduce Attrition

Retention can be dramatically impacted by patient satisfaction with aspects of the study or investigative site. A routine patient satisfaction assessment process identifies specific sources of dissatisfaction and addresses them before it's too late. The dissatisfaction can be very minor or appear almost trivial to the site staff but the importance to the participant should not be made light of. These items can be: the availability of parking, the waiting room temperature, the boredom of the waiting caregiver, availability of refreshments or the infrequency of hearing the words "thank you."

Reinforcement

Reinforcement can be executed through simple but recurrent efforts on the part of the sites to keep the study "top of mind" with the participants. Examples are:

- A year's membership in a support group or national association for their disease such as the National Osteoporosis Foundation or the American Heart Association
- A calendar for the study with appointment reminder stickers
- Kept appointment "Thank You" letters from the Investigator
- Birthday and Holiday Cards
- A study-focused newsletter
- Educational materials gathered from credible, independent sources on exercise, nutrition and disease-specific tips for "total health"
- Group activities at the site such as lectures, book clubs, cooking tips, local support group meetings
- Customer Service Desk
  - Toll-free number available for participants if they have a complaint about the study and do not wish to directly talk to the site about it
  - Hours of operations would be Monday through Friday 9AM to 8PM ET
  - After-hours callers would be able to leave a voice mail message for a return call the next business day

Table 4: Retention Challenges and Opportunities

Key Issues in Clinical Trials	Possible Solutions
1. Critical elements of adherence in randomized clinical trials are often not addressed	– Tailored communication support driven by patient needs leads to a better patient experience/improved results
2. Staff and investigators often don't understand the importance of adherence and retention	– Self-training tools – Retention guidelines – "What to do" instructions for Investigator site staff to address patients at risk of dropout
3. Cues to non-adherence often surface during the descriptive consent period	– Pre-screener designed to pick up cues to non-adherence and select highest scoring prospects
4. Study participants often join a trial to obtain "treatment"; randomization is a disappointment if not well understood	– Communicate concept clearly – Provide "health-oriented" benefit that both test and control participants will receive
5. Opportunity to collect adherence data is often overlooked by investigators	– Initiate centralized tracking of patient non-adherence cues – Set up feedback loop from investigative sites and patients regarding progress
6. Rewards, recognition and appreciation are tools proven to be effective at driving ongoing participation, though non-relevant incentives can have a negative impact	– Tailoring and monitoring software enables incentives to be made more meaningful to the patient
7. Recovering dropouts or improving poor adherence requires burdensome administration by investigative sites	– Automated process and centralized support to handle these duties saves time and money, improves efficiency

8. Participant attrition has been directly correlated with number and timing of follow-up contacts

— Reduce inconvenience to patient and maintain relationships by centralizing and automating follow-up communications that are consistent with study objectives and fill the gaps between visits

9. Participants are more likely to be committed to a long-term study if they can identify and describe it

— Brand study with a patient-friendly identity that is meaningful and impactful

10. A multimedia approach can help participants understand study requirements

— Explanatory audio and video can be provided to patients via audiotapes, videotapes or the web

11. Application of a participant tracking strategy is underutilized in the design of many trials—and is too sensitive to be left to chance at the investigative site level

— A centralized database in a HIPAA-compliant environment allows specific tracking of progress and study participants

12. Retention can be dramatically impacted by patient satisfaction with aspects of study or investigative site

— A patient satisfaction assessment process identifies specific sources of dissatisfaction and addresses them before it's too late

13. Patients join studies to improve their own health as well as to contribute to science

— Provide a "study mission" communication early in the process to reinforce patient's commitment to the trial's purpose

— Deliver outcomes studies and reports to document predictors or "drivers" of compliance and recruitment success (contributing to the science of trial management)

Appreciation Items

While many sponsors are sensitive about the concept of providing "gifts" to participants, appreciation items can be utilized to expand patients' knowledge of their disease or to make their participation in the study a bit easier. Some of the items used in the past have all been less than $25 in value and are only offered for a particular event such as a milestone in the study.

Examples are:

- A tote bag to carry the patient's diary, unused medication, papers, bottled water, etc.
- Books about their disease or helpful guidelines for their caregiver
- Flowers, movie theater passes or similar items at the halfway point of their participation

Summary

Nothing can replace the power of genuine concern by the site personnel, creating for the participant a feeling of belonging to some worthwhile cause, showing respect, gratitude and listening. Recruitment, retention and compliance efforts need the human touch to be successful and these can only be done at "the point of care." Participants are more likely to be committed to a long-term study if they can identify and describe it.

Key Takeaways

- The foundation for a patient communication program begins with research.
- Participant commitment is never greater than at the time of recruitment.
- Establish a trusting and tolerant relationship to foster compliance.
- Involve a third party for support such as spouse, friend or relative.
- Discuss retention and adherence techniques that will be utilized and the frequency of contact.
- Utilize positive reinforcement for compliance successes.
- Provide current and relevant information on disease for the patient and caregiver.
- Discuss study design challenges as early as possible.
- Present the benefits of finishing study.
- Discuss the value of trials to the general public.

Author Biography

John Needham

John Needham has 28 years of experience in the fields of market development, healthcare relationship marketing, patient accrual, compliance and retention. John was Co-Founder and President of Alliance Marketing Services Group, a firm specializing in the development and implementation of direct marketing programs in health care. In addition, he was the General Manager and Co-Founder of PatientQuest, a clinical trial recruiting and retention firm. He has served in senior management positions at Telerx Marketing, TeleSpectrum Worldwide, PharmaKinetics Laboratories, Acurian and Pepsi Cola USA.

John also serves as a Captain in the United States Naval Reserve.

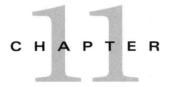

Community, Physician and Consumer Outreach Strategies to Meet Recruitment Goals

Diana L. Anderson, Ph.D., D. Anderson & Company

Objectives
- Establish community outreach as an effective recruitment tool.
- Identify the many types of community outreach activities.
- Differentiate between short-term techniques designed to enhance enrollment of currently enrolling clinical trials, and longer-term approaches aimed at educating consumers and physicians about clinical research in general.
- Raise awareness that different methods of community outreach may be needed to recruit traditionally underrepresented groups in clinical trials, such as minorities, elderly, women and children.

Introduction

Creating public awareness of clinical trials is key to meeting enrollment targets. Multi-faceted central campaigns that drive recruitment are growing in popularity, and they can also be costly.

One promotional technique that is gaining recognition is quite possibly the most obvious and the least expensive—community outreach. Millions of dollars may be spent annually on advertising and corporate sponsorships, but for building trust and capitalizing on the targeted audience, there is no substitute for reaching out to the local community. Getting involved can increase the visibility of an investigative site while at the same time, enhance its reputation as a socially responsible and caring member of the community with much to offer.

Spreading the word about clinical trials in a community setting is critical to the reaching of enrollment goals because despite the millions spent on media advertising, a large majority of Americans do not know what a clinical trial is and are unaware of studies going on in their communities. In a recent survey of more than 1,000 adults, nearly three-quarters of respondents, 74%, reported having very limited knowledge of clinical research.[1] This may explain why a mere 10% of adult Americans have participated in clinical trials.[2]

Yet, if asked or given the opportunity, 77% stated in a different survey that they would consider participating.[3] Only 16% of respondents claimed to have had an opportunity to consider participation in clinical trials. As these data highlight, reaching out to prospective study volunteers through community initiatives may be a good way for sites to inform them about clinical trials in general, while piquing their interest in specific trials for which they might qualify.

Reaching Out to the Community

Community outreach refers to involvement in activities for the purpose of creating public awareness of the various clinical research opportunities taking place in the local community. Similar to a central recruitment campaign, which is often a multi-media endeavor, the community outreach effort also

---

Table 1: Community Outreach Techniques

- Contact local and national chapters of professional organizations such as American Diabetes Association, American Heart Association, etc.

- Contact support groups, community centers, and county hospitals

- Mail attractive, professional-looking mailers to physicians, pharmacists, and direct mail databases, and follow up with telephone calls

- Develop disease-/indication-specific web sites

- Offer health forums such as lunch-and-learn sessions

- Participate in local health fairs

- Sponsor local walks for breast cancer, Alzheimer's disease, AIDS, etc.

- Contact local TV and radio health reporters about ongoing studies

- Keep metrics on success of various initiatives

---

tends to be multi-faceted. It involves networking with professional organizations, patient advocacy support groups, community centers, physicians and pharmacists. It can take the form of participating in health fairs, sponsoring the local breast cancer walk, conducting free diabetes screening, hosting lunch-and-learn events, or volunteering on the board of local chapters of various disease organizations such as arthritis, Alzheimer's, lupus, etc. (see Table 1). These activities help clinical professionals create awareness of their site and its ongoing studies while networking with the targeted audience.

According to social theory, individuals seek to connect with one or more communities to form sustainable and beneficial relationships that last over time. In forming these relationships, the individual is better positioned to further his or her personal goals, and the community benefits from the talents offered by the many individuals making up the community. This instinct for community is seen throughout the animal kingdom, not just in human society.[4]

Applying the "need for community" theory to the practical aspects of patient recruitment means identifying how an investigative site can best meet the needs of prospective study volunteers while reaching its enrollment goals. Research suggests that prospective subjects have needs that affect their willingness to participate in clinical trials (see Table 2).[5] Altruism (advancing medicine, helping others), and personal interests (earning extra money, obtaining better treatment for conditions) are key motivators so it behooves investigative sites to try to meet those needs.

Table 2: Reasons for Participation in Clinical Research (n=2,023 adults)

■ To advance medicine/science	54%
■ To help others with the condition	46%
■ To earn extra money	42%
■ To obtain better treatment for my condition	40%
■ Education about treatment/improving my health	37%
■ Information read, seen or heard about the study	36%
■ Doctor recommended the study	25%
■ Curiosity about study/medical practice	23%
■ To obtain free medication	24%
■ Had a life-threatening illness	5%

Source: Harris Interactive Survey, May 2003

Nanette Myers, Director of Patient Recruitment at D. Anderson & Co., says that in designing an initiative that meets the needs of prospective subjects, and ultimately leads to enrollment, she first considers how to find and establish a rapport with the targeted audience. Once that is accomplished, the next step is to build a relationship, so when another study for the same therapeutic indication comes along, the relationship is already in place.

Myers says a good place to begin building rapport is with professional organizations. "We often start by mailing IRB[institutional review board]-approved information about our enrolling studies to national and local chapters of the professional organizations, such as the American Diabetes Association, or the National Arthritis Foundation. Then, we follow up with a phone call to see what kinds of information or services we can provide," Myers says.

Local chapters are sometimes seeking speakers for regularly scheduled programs. This presents an opportunity for a local investigative site to have face-to-face contact by providing a speaker, either an investigator or a study coordinator, for lunch-and-learn sessions or dinner meetings for an interested audience. Myers adds, "At local meetings, it is sometimes possible to screen people right there."

In addition to contacting professional organizations, Myers explains that establishing a rapport with the many free clinics in the United States can be a valuable source of referrals. "This is particularly true when recruiting for certain indications, such as Type 2 diabetes, which is one of the top therapeutic areas under study today. Because of the increasing prevalence of the disease and the demographics of who is at greater risk of developing Type 2 diabetes, you realize that free clinics are a good choice," says Myers.

Free clinics are sometimes interested in scheduling a diabetes educator or an investigator to speak in a public forum about the disease, and when this happens, the recruiting company can provide refreshments, literature about diabetes and information about ongoing studies. Oftentimes, the sponsor is willing to provide useful giveaways such as pens, or sticky notes, t-shirts or caps.

County hospitals tend to have large support groups for a variety of therapeutic indications, and reaching out to them for recruitment purposes can be productive, once rapport has been established. Local investigative sites may have already developed a relationship with the local county hospital, so in that instance, it may be more effective for the site to use its contacts at that institution to promote awareness of enrolling studies of interest. Taking this approach is probably faster and more productive than relying on an outside patient recruitment firm to first contact the hospital, and then go through the preliminary steps of finding the right person, and then begin establishing a rapport. Using the local site's already established contacts is an approach that can be used in numerous venues.

Other methods of community outreach include creating a study-specific Web site, and contacting religious organizations, patient advocacy groups or community centers that may have access to special populations such as ethnic minority groups and seniors. In addition, when targeting seniors, retirement communities can be contacted. Information and posters can be mailed out, and then followed up with a phone call and an offer to give a presentation.

Table 3: Sample Poster

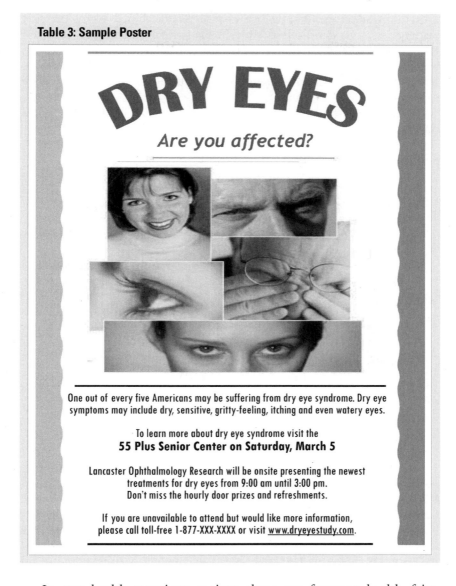

In our health-conscious society, there are frequent health fairs. Hospitals, non-profit organizations, corporations, municipalities, schools and universities sponsor these events with regularity and they seek quality exhibitors to inform the public about the ever-changing healthcare field. This venue can be used to educate people about clinical trials, the role of the investigative site and how the individual might participate.

Investigative sites might consider sponsoring a booth at a health fair. The booth should be decorated to look as inviting as possible. Attractive posters and literature should be neatly displayed and refreshments might be used as a draw. In addition, offering free cholesterol-screenings, blood pressure readings, or bone density tests are valuable services that attract passersby. Employees representing the site are its ambassadors and should be friendly, well groomed, identified with a name badge that identifies his or her position along with the company name and be genuinely interested in providing information.

Metrics suggest that health fairs can offer a particularly effective one-on-one contact between a possibly interested study volunteer and a caring representative from the investigative site (see Table 4). For this reason, health fairs can yield a good return on investment.

Table 4: Results of Community Outreach Efforts for a Diabetes Study

Initiative	Total # Attended/ Mailed To	Referred to Study	Scheduled	DNQ*	Consented
Health Fairs	12,938	875	40	28	12
Patient Mailings	1,115	20	8	0	8
Education Classes	239	5	3	2	3
Physician Mailings	2,187	1	0	1	0
ADA Sponsorship	4,650	3	0	0	0
Community Mailings	1,520	2	0	0	0
Total	**23,348**	**906**	**51**	**31**	**23**

* DNQ = did not qualify

Source: D. Anderson & Co.

Tom Calzone, Director of Operations for Rochester Clinical Research in Rochester, New York, agrees that face-to-face contact can be highly effective. Calzone explains that his investigative site invites the public in for a free diabetes screening, using a finger-prick technique, followed by a blood pressure reading. He says, "Once or twice a month, I place information in local newspapers announcing the free screening. The copy has been reviewed by an IRB, although it is not necessarily connected to any specific study."

The site schedules the appointments; dedicates staff, often two nurses; and as many as forty patients may be scheduled. Results are explained to the patient and sent to the person's primary care physician. According to Calzone, "From the forty screens, it's not unusual for the site to end up enrolling two or three patients in ongoing diabetes trials."

The screenings are really about building rapport with the community. Information on enrolling studies is displayed at the site, but Calzone has learned that prospective subjects generally do not want to hear about clinical studies right away. At first, they are more comfortable asking questions about what the site does, and what a clinical trial is. "When I first started the free screenings in 2002, I had only one intention, to enroll people in studies. We quickly learned that pushing the studies too hard turns people off, especially when you are advertising a free screening. Since then, we have softened our approach, and decided to just offer the free screenings, and approach the subject when the person's blood sugar might qualify them to enter one of several diabetes studies," says Calzone.

If someone's blood sugar seems to be seriously out of control, the nurse suggests the individual see his or her doctor immediately, and the site may schedule a free half-hour session with a registered dietician. Calzone says that it sends a positive message when a site is offering these types of quality services at no cost to the consumer.

Jay Udani, M.D., Medical Director of Pacific West Research in Northridge, Calif., says that his investigative site offers various types of community outreach based on educating the public about various health topics, first, and providing information about clinical trials, second. Udani comments, "I give lectures to the lay public at least twice a month and through this educational process, I've learned that it is important to establish a rapport first with people before broaching the subject of clinical trials."

Table 5: Tips for a Successful Health Forum

- Identify a speaker and check availability.

- Mail invitations to a targeted audience. Advertise through public service announcements, newspapers and flyers. Always include an invitation to the press.

- Reserve a location in advance. Hospitals and municipal centers are excellent choices and are rarely expensive.

- Decide on the format of the event. Will you provide refreshments, door prizes, and screenings?

- Provide questionnaires, giveaways, fliers on clinical trials, and on enrolling in upcoming studies.

- Capture names and addresses of those who attend these events and be prepared to screen individuals who express interest in specific studies.

- The scope of the event will depend on your individual budget, but consider approaching the pharmaceutical sponsor of the studies for which you are trying to recruit.

- Avoid holiday time and months when the weather is severe.

- Send a follow-up thank you letter with a list of upcoming studies that you think would be of interest to them.

Udani says he ends his lectures by providing information about the latest advances, and then segues into the fact that research is ongoing, and that Pacific West is offering the opportunity to participate. "After the lecture, if you have an opportunity to talk with someone one-on-one, and then bring up the research, they are more amenable to the idea than if your first contact with them is about the research," says Udani.

Health forums about a specific disease, such as the ones conducted by Pacific West, can be effective tools for increasing enrollment. They are usually conducted by a specialist in that field and are open to an invited audience or to the public. Successful health forums take careful planning to increase the likelihood of a good turnout. When planning a forum, consider the points listed in Table 5.

Long Range Outreach

Community outreach can be thought of as having short-term and long-range goals. Short-term community outreach has the immediate purpose of enhancing patient enrollment for currently ongoing studies. Longer-range objectives have the broader intent of educating the public about clinical trials in general, and informing interested parties about where they can find information about specific studies if they seek participation for themselves, or for family or friends. Udani of Pacific West Research would like pharmaceutical sponsors to take a leading role in public education campaigns with a fervor similar to what they exhibit in their direct-to-consumer advertising programs. Udani explains, "If the same degree of effort were applied toward getting people to understand clinical trials, more people would be driven into their doctors' offices to ask about possible participation. This type of initiative could possibly transform the consumer into someone who is interested in being screened, or possibly enrolled."

Organized public education campaigns aimed at increasing awareness of clinical research and currently enrolling trials could prove to be a more effective recruitment method than the current approach that many prospective study volunteers use—relying on their physicians to advise them about clinical trials. According to a survey of some 1,000 adults, 73% of prospective candidates want their physicians involved in the decision to participate in a study, and 51% want their physician involved if they ultimately enroll.[6]

Yet, the disconnect for potential subjects who rely on their physicians to help them make informed decisions about enrollment is that the vast majority of physicians do not participate in clinical trials and may know little or nothing about which ones are ongoing, or where patients can find reliable information. According to the American Medical Association, there are approximately 836,000 physicians in the United States,[7] and of those, a mere 35,000, or 4%, file a Form FDA 1572 annually.[8]

This minimal amount of physician involvement may at least partially explain why millions of adult Americans, some 73 million, are turning to the Internet to seek health information, with six million searching on a typical day.[9] According to a 2002 survey conducted by the Pew Internet Project, of the 73 million health information seekers, 48% are seeking information about alternative or experimental treatments or medicines. This fact bodes well for the various web sites that provide information about ongoing studies (see Table 6) and attests to the strong public interest that could be tapped for clinical research.

Table 6: A Sampling of Clinical Trials Web Sites

- www.acurian.com
- http://cancer.gov/clinicaltrials
- www.cc.nih.gov
- www.centerwatch.com
- www.clinicaltrials.com
- www.clinicaltrials.gov
- www.emergingmed.com
- www.trialscentral.org/index.html
- www.veritasmedicine.com

Source: Harris Interactive Survey, May 2003

Similar to what has been reported in other surveys about patients' strong trust in their own physicians, the Pew survey cautions that web surfers still seek to discuss with their physicians the information found online. Only a small percentage of survey participants, 18%, said they would substitute online information for advice from their own physicians.

Because patients maintain continued reliance on their doctor's judgment, an outreach effort to inform physicians about clinical research is strongly indicated. Long-range community outreach may include exploring ways to interest more physicians and physicians-in-training in the clinical development process so they are better prepared to help prospective study volunteers evaluate appropriate trials.

Greater physician awareness of clinical trials will also serve industry's needs to boost the number of physicians interested in becoming investigators or referral sources of volunteers, if the number of patients needed per new drug application (NDA) is to be met. Current estimates place the number of evaluable patients needed per NDA in excess of 5,000,[10] a number that is growing faster than the volume of physicians willing to become investigators.[11] There is a projected 15% shortfall in the number of investigators needed by 2005.[12]

Mark Ridge, Manager of Clinical Recruitment Support at Centocor, says that his company recognizes the importance of reaching out to both physicians and consumers, and is taking preliminary steps to educate both groups about clinical trials in general, and about specific studies that are taking place around the globe. "We created a tool kit that our investigators can use to reach out to other physicians and patients in their communities for an ulcerative colitis project that is taking place in 140 sites worldwide," Ridge explains. "The kit includes a number of materials: an educational brochure about clinical trials; another about specific trials and the time commitment involved; sticky notes to flag the charts of patients who could possibly qualify for the study; flyers about clinical trials that can be posted in physician breakrooms; and a physician referral letter on a CD-ROM that an investigator can easily personalize and send out to community physicians along with a small pocket card that lists the criteria for study inclusion."

According to Ridge, preliminary feedback has been quite positive, including some comments that this sort of comprehensive outreach approach should become standard practice. At the time of this writing, there are no metrics to document the success of the program basically for two reasons: the initiative is new, and, also, it is difficult to document which patients are the direct result of this effort because the idea is for Centocor Investigators to reach out to physicians in the community, most of whom are not Centocor Investigators, and therefore, have no reason to document referrals.

Ridge says that despite the lack of clear-cut metrics, and specific return-on-investment (ROI) data, there is no doubt that enrollment is increasing. And perhaps more importantly, this community outreach effort will go a long way toward educating the community and physicians about clinical trials, and going forward will motivate both groups to consider participation as a reasonable choice for potential volunteers, and patient referral as a reasonable choice for physicians.

Carol Alter, co-founder of Frontier Medical Research, says this company is developing tele-recruiting, a model that actively involves community-based primary care physicians in the referral process by linking their offices to dedicated clinical research sites. Tele-recruiting creates a link using tele-video equipment that Frontier places in the office of the primary care physician. According to Alter, "If a patient is identified as possibly meeting criteria for a study, either by chart review, or during an office visit, the referring physician can advise the patient of the study, and if he or she is interested, the doctor can walk that patient to the room containing the televideo equipment, the study or 'core' site is called, and at that moment, the study coordinator can schedule an appointment for the prospective candidate. Also, if a primary care practice is sufficiently large, it could possibly accommodate tel-erecruiting links to more than one core site."

Metrics from an osteoarthritis study show the effectiveness of tele-recruiting, which involves the patient's physician in a face-to-face interaction, vs. conventional call center response (see Table 7).

Table 7: Recruiting for an Osteoarthritis Study

Frontier Medical Process		National Ad Campaign	
Number of patients eligible at prescreen	37	Number of patients referred from call center	30
Number of patients agreeing to telerecruitment screening	13	Number of appropriate patients to go to willing investigative site for screen	20
Number of patients meeting criteria at screening	10		
Number of patients seen at core site and enrolled	10	Number of patients enrolled in study	2
Time required	3 weeks @ 10 hrs/week	Time required by research staff	6 weeks @ 20 hrs/week

Alter says that if the core site is not conveniently located for the study candidate, the system has the capability to allow the patient to participate in the study remotely. "All study visits would be done through the telemedicine device, yet all of the study data would reside at the core site. Currently, we are validating a number of processes that would allow this to happen, and several pharmaceutical Sponsors have expressed interest in this capability," Alter comments.

Formal Physician Training and Other Long-Term Investments

To tap into the number of doctors needed to become either investigators or referral sources, it may be productive for organizations within the pharmaceutical industry, or the sponsors themselves, to consider long-term solutions such as formal education campaigns to teach more physicians about what clinical trials are, what good clinical practice (GCP) is and how to participate as investigators. This proactive technique could mitigate, at least to some degree, long-standing problems linked to inadequate patient databases, missed enrollment targets and the moving of patient recruitment into rescue mode.

At the time of this writing, three organizations, the American Academy of Pharmaceutical Physicians (AAPP), the Association of Clinical Research Professionals (ACRP) and the Drug Information Association (DIA) are structuring programs to teach interested physicians the many guidelines that govern clinical investigation. The purpose of the programs is to provide investigators with basic knowledge of the regulations and of their responsibilities, the critical importance of protecting study participants and the ethics involved in conducting clinical research (see Table 8).

Table 8: Programs to Train Clinical Investigators

Organization	Type of Program	Scope
American Academy of Pharmaceutical Physicians (AAPP) (www.aapp.org)	Examination leads to Certified Physician Investigator (CPI) designation	Four domains of learning: - Comply with regulations - Protect study participants - Conduct the study - Manage study site
Association of Clinical Research Professionals (ACRP) (www.acrpnet.org)	Examination leads to Certified Clinical Research Investigator (CCRI) designation	Three key areas: - GCP-compliance - Practical aspects of conducting clinical trials - Drug development and test design module
Drug Information Association (DIA) (www.diahome.org)	Examination leads to Certified Clinical Investigator (CCI) designation	Three key areas: - Roles and responsibilities - Regulations and guidelines governing clinical investigation - Practices that ensure effective and efficient study conduct

Beth Harper, Senior Vice President of Operations at RRI, believes that in addition to Investigator training courses offered by various organizations, other outreach techniques may include industry-sponsored scholarship programs, or mentoring programs. "Medical students could be sponsored to receive training in clinical research, and as part of the program, after completion of training, these doctors, could work in underserved areas. This approach would enable these doctors to establish relationships with populations that, so far, have been difficult to reach. This sort of industry-sponsored training could be seen as a long-term investment," says Harper.

Industry has started to make long-term investments by collaborating with government and academic investigators to improve patient recruitment in early stage cancer trials. One of the first such public-private partnerships launched in July 2003 and grew out of the recognition that the vast majority of cancer patients are not made aware of clinical trials. In a recent survey of 6,000 cancer patients, 85% of them reported that they either did not know about clinical trials or were not sure that they were an option, yet 75% of them reported willingness to enroll had they known that it was possible to do so.[13]

In an effort to improve this statistic, five pharmaceutical firms—Aventis, Bristol-Myers Squibb, Eli Lilly and Company, GlaxoSmithKline and Novartis—came together with the National Cancer Institute and the Foundation for the National Institutes of Health to put forth $5.7 million to be awarded to six cancer centers (see Table 9). The goal of the initiative is for the six centers to use the grants to design and implement new approaches to increase access to phase I and II clinical trials for as many people as possible, with special emphasis on increasing minority and geriatric participation by removing barriers to access.[14]

Table 9: Cancer Centers Receiving Funding to Reach Out Especially to Minority and Geriatric Populations

- Massachusetts General Hospital
- Ohio State University Comprehensive Cancer Center
- University of California, Davis
- University of Colorado Health Science Center
- University of Pittsburgh Cancer Institute
- Washington University, St. Louis

Source: Foundation for the National Institutes of Health, www.nih.org

---

According to the Foundation for the National Institutes of Health, proposed methodology for success might include online protocol information, development of culturally relevant literature about the incidence of various types of cancer and a budget allowance for travel and day care services for prospective enrollees. Some of the institutions might consider developing a community-based model whereby volunteers can visit community-based oncologists instead of traveling to a somewhat intimidating or possibly more distant major medical center.

At the time of this writing, this initiative is just launching, so metrics are not available as to the success of the plan.

Reaching Out to Special Populations

Oftentimes, the most carefully orchestrated outreach strategies are not enough to attract sufficient numbers of special populations such as African-Americans, Latinos, elderly, children, even women. Chapter 13 of this book is dedicated to the subject of recruiting special populations, but in light of its obvious connection to community outreach efforts, a few key highlights are presented here.

Different tactics are needed to reach out to difficult-to-recruit populations, as seen in the collaborative cancer trials outreach program involving government, industry and academic medical centers. For these segments of the population, the building of a trusting relationship between a prospective volunteer and the healthcare provider is perhaps the single most effective route to increasing enrollment.

Doug Miller, M.D., Professor of Medicine and Associate Director of Division of Geriatric Medicine at St. Louis University, says that when it comes to reaching out to minority and/or older populations, the place to start is by demonstrating a strong commitment to the community by getting involved in local health issues and delivering quality health services. Through this connection of community-based service, a genuine level of trust can develop slowly over time, and according to James Powell, M.D., Director of Biomedical Education and Research for the National Medical Association (NMA), when trying to recruit underrepresented sub-populations, there is no substitute for creating a sense of trustworthiness.

Dr. Powell adds that in the African-American community, anecdotal data suggest that the recruitment process is most successful when there is a cultural concordance between the patient and the physician. "To achieve this success, that is, to get better representation of minority patients, it's important to get minority physicians involved," Powell says.

To move toward that goal, the National Medical Association, through a grant from the Department of Health and Human Services/Office of Minority Health, launched Project IMPACT in 2000. An acronym for Increase Minority Participation and Awareness of Clinical Trials, Project IMPACT was designed to educate minority physicians and consumers about the potential benefits of participating in clinical trials. Through this effort, validity of clinical data supporting the safe and effective use of various therapies in African-American patients would, hopefully, be improved. The decision to move forward with Project IMPACT followed conclusions drawn by an NMA consensus panel that the lack of clinical trial participation by minorities could potentially contribute to health disparities because not enough is known about the impact of certain therapies on the African-American population.

Project IMPACT training programs have been ongoing across the country for the past few years, both for physicians and consumers. Some physicians receive an intensive two-day training designed to prepare them to become investigators, or help them advise their patients about participation in clinical trials. Through "You've Got the Power," the consumer portion of Project IMPACT, the community learns about clinical trials through a variety of means, such as health fairs, and presentations at organizational conferences and community meetings.

At the time of this writing, NMA is about to embark on a survey of physicians who have completed Project IMPACT training to determine their current level of involvement in the clinical research process. No data are yet available to evaluate the project's success on minority recruitment in clinical trials.

Inclusion of minorities and various underrepresented groups in clinical research is strongly encouraged by the National Institutes of Health and FDA. The Agency has long requested race and ethnicity data on subjects in certain clinical trials, as evidenced by the numerous guidances issued on the subject. In a new draft guidance, *Collection of Race and Ethnicity Data in Clinical Trials*, the FDA is now making recommendations on the categories to use when collecting and reporting those data.[15] The draft guidance does not require an increased number of participants or members of underrepresented groups but rather represents the agency's current thinking on how to collect race and ethnicity data in clinical trials. The Agency is also encouraging, and in some cases, requiring testing of investigational compounds in children and elderly (see Table 10).

Government's interest in including diverse populations in clinical trials, to better evaluate the safety and effectiveness of investigational compounds and devices, spurs community outreach efforts to reach these groups.

Table 10: Government Efforts to Encourage Inclusion of Underrepresented Populations in Clinical Research

1989	Guideline for the Study of Drugs Likely to Be Used in the Elderly (FDA)
1993	NIH Revitalization Act—directed NIH to establish guidelines for including women and minorities in NIH-sponsored research
	Guideline for the Study and Evaluation of Gender Differences in the Clinical Evaluation of Drugs (FDA)
1998	FDA Demographic Rule requiring sponsors to tabulate the numbers of participants in clinical trials by age group, gender and race
2001	Content and Format for Geriatric Labeling (FDA)
2002	Best Pharmaceuticals for Children Act
2003	Collection of Race and Ethnicity Data in Clinical Trials, FDA Draft Guidance
	Pediatric Research Equity Act

Source: www.fda.gov

Community Outreach Review

As the pressure to reach enrollment targets becomes ever more intense, it behooves investigative sites and sponsors to pursue multiple avenues to reach out to the community. Advertising dollars can be used very effectively to stimulate interest for currently enrolling trials, but the aim of community outreach should be greater than reaching short term recruitment goals. From the site's perspective, community outreach efforts should increase visibility of the site, develop a positive image and establish rapport with the community, all in an effort to increase awareness of ongoing trials and the clinical research process.

There are many ways to get the message out, both for the purposes of meeting enrollment targets for ongoing studies, and for general education. Health fairs, direct mail, health forums, local fundraising walks for diseases such as breast cancer or diabetes, free screenings, establishing study-specific web sites, and contacting local radio and TV stations are just some of the many possible approaches. Following each community contact, metrics can be kept to document the techniques that prove most successful.

Experienced sites have learned that when engaging in these community activities, people respond more favorably to the idea of clinical research when they are first educated about their disease of interest and presented with information about a specific study, second. Discussions about ongoing studies should wait until the site has taken the time to establish a rapport. High pressure recruitment tactics are rarely successful.

Raising awareness should have a long-term positive impact on recruitment as various surveys have revealed that a large percentage of Americans, 74%, have little or no knowledge of clinical trials. For cancer patients, the numbers are even higher, approximately 85%, yet many of those respondents state that they would be interested in clinical trials if made aware of them. This lack of familiarity explains why so few Americans, about 10%, have participated in clinical studies to date.

In addition to educating the public, it is critical to educate more physicians about clinical research. Despite the volume of clinical trial information easily available on the Internet, research suggests that patients still prefer to discuss study participation with their physicians. Unfortunately, very few doctors know about studies of potential interest, and even fewer, some 4%, are clinical investigators. While there are no specific numbers to document how many doctors refer patients to trials, the number is believed to be low.

For this reason, a broad-based education campaign targeting physicians that focuses on the specifics of clinical trials and the responsibilities of investigators is indicated. Several organizations, such as the American Academy of Pharmaceutical Physicians, Association of Clinical Research Professionals and the Drug Information Association, have launched training courses that will certify physicians who take courses and pass examinations. In addition, various sponsors and industry providers are reaching out to the physician community to increase their awareness of ongoing trials.

Ideally, physician education campaigns would take place alongside ones aimed at consumers. That way, as consumers learn about clinical research, more of them may present at their doctors' offices, seeking advice, and those doctors would be able to respond more knowledgeably as to the appropriateness of certain trials for their patients.

Minority populations have long been recognized as being underrepresented in clinical research, due largely to suspicion of the process, often as a result of past abuses. Anecdotal information suggests that key elements to successful minority recruiting are trust between the physician and patient, and similarity in ethnic background between physician and patient. In recognition of these recruitment factors, initiatives designed to reach out to minority physicians and patients, such as public-private-academic collaborations, and Project IMPACT Sponsored by the National Medical Association (NMA), hold the promise of increasing recruitment.

These efforts and others reflect the government's continuing interest in casting a wider net to recruit underrepresented sub-populations such as minorities, elderly, women and children. Devising ways to reach these groups is critical for collecting data suggestive of appropriate dosages for various ages, ethnic groups and gender.

Community outreach is an effective way to connect individuals with the clinical trials process. It also serves their altruistic interests and offers the opportunity to seek help for their medical conditions. Community outreach is an important complement to advertising campaigns because it has the capacity to affect people in a personal way.

Key Takeaways

- Successful community outreach is about establishing a rapport with prospective volunteers. This approach allows them to become comfortable with the idea of participating in clinical research.
- To establish the necessary rapport, the investigative site can offer a host of activities that educate consumers about various diseases of interest. Provide education first, and broach the subject of clinical research second.
- There is a serious lack of awareness and understanding of clinical research among the general population and a lack of participation in clinical research by physicians. Long-term community outreach efforts are needed to educate consumers and physicians about clinical research.
- Various professional organizations have established training programs to teach physicians about the regulatory and ethical aspects of becoming clinical Investigators.
- Successful recruiting of traditionally underrepresented groups, such as minorities, elderly, women and children, requires techniques that create a strong degree of trust between the individual and the Investigator.

Research suggests that minorities tend to be most comfortable with Investigators of a similar ethnic background.

- FDA has put forth a number of guidances for industry directed at improving representation of minorities, elderly, women and children in clinical research.

References

1. *Op. cit.*, "Improving Recruitment and Retention Practices Based on Input from the Public and Patients."
2. *The Many Reasons Why People Do (and Would) Participate in Clinical Trials*, Harris Interactive, June 16, 2003.
3. Ibid., *The Many Reasons Why People Do (and Would) Participate in Clinical Trials*.
4. *The Community of the Future*, Frances Hesselbein, editor, et. al., Jossey-Bass, Inc., 1998, p. 10.
5. *The Many Reasons Why People Do (and Would) Participate in Clinical Trials*, Harris Interactive, June 16, 2003.
6. Interactive Volunteer Study, Ken Getz, CenterWatch and Illumina Interactive, November 2002.
7. AMA Total Physicians by Race/Ethnicity—2001, www.ama-assn.org, accessed August 8, 2003.
8. DataEdge, FDA, 2001.
9. *Vital Decisions: How Internet users decide what information to trust when they or loved ones are sick*, Pew Internet & American Life, May 2002, www.pewinternet.org/reports/pdfs/PIP_Vital_Decisions_May2002.pdf.
10. Tufts Center for the Study of Drug Development, 2002.
11. *Patient Recruitment: The growing challenge for pharmaceutical companies*, IBM Global Industries, June 2002, p. 3.
12. "Anticipating a Clinical Investigator Shortfall", *CenterWatch*, April 2001.
13. *Misconceptions and Lack of Awareness Greatly Reduce Recruitment for Cancer Clinical Trials*, Harris Interactive, January 22, 2001.
14. *NIH-Pharmaceutical Industry Partnership Announces First Grants for Overcoming Barriers to Early Phase Clinical Trials: Unique Collaboration Assists Six Cancer Centers Across U.S.*, Foundation for the National Institutes of Health, www.fnih.org, July 9, 2003.
15. Draft Guidance for Industry on the Collection of Race and Ethnicity Data in Clinical Trials for FDA Regulated Products, Federal Register, Vol. 68, No. 20, January 30, 2003, www.fda.gov/OHRMS/DOCKETS/98fr/5054dft.doc

Author Biography

Diana L. Anderson, Ph.D.
President and CEO, D. L. Anderson International, Inc.

Dr. Diana L. Anderson is the President, CEO and Founder of D. L. Anderson International, Inc., parent company to subsidiaries D. Anderson & Company, a patient recruitment provider and RRI, a Contract Research Organization. D. Anderson & Company, the patient recruitment arm of D. L. Anderson International, Inc., provides a comprehensive menu of specialized services to the clinical trials industry. These services include consulting and patient recruitment management, market research and feasibility assessments, media management and purchasing, creative development, regulatory management, clinical trial branding, community outreach and public relations, site-specific recruitment services, direct-to-consumer strategies, call center support and retention programs.

Dr. Anderson consults globally as a recognized authority in the field of patient recruitment, with recent presentations in Japan, Europe and Israel. She is widely published and frequently featured for her accomplishments in a variety of trade publications and scientific journals. She is also the author of the books *50 Ways to Cope with Arthritis, A Guide to Patient Recruitment* and *A Guide to Patient Recruitment and Retention.*

Dr. Anderson serves on several corporate boards and in various capacities on committees including Immediate Past Chair of the Association of Clinical Research Professionals (ACRP). She has previously held appointments on the Board of Directors of the North Texas Chapter of the Arthritis Foundation; Editorial Board, Arthritis Today Magazine; Past President, Association of Rheumatology Health Professionals (ARHP); Board of Trustees of the National Arthritis Foundation; Board of Directors, American College of Rheumatology; and Past President, Western U.S.A. Pain Society. She maintains memberships and remains actively involved in a number of these professional organizations.

She holds a Ph.D. from Texas Woman's University, M.S.N. from the University of Texas Health Care Science Center in San Antonio, Texas, and a B.S.N. from the University of Nebraska.

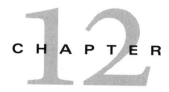

CHAPTER

Customer Service in Clinical Trials: Making the Patient Experience Meaningful and Memorable

Steve Wishnack, Think & Do™

Objectives

- Create awareness of the need for applying customer service to clinical trials.
- Demonstrate the value of creating a customer-centered culture within sponsor and investigative site organizations.
- Share principles of customer service that can have a positive impact on patient recruitment and retention for clinical trials.
- Suggest ways to integrate effective customer service in the clinical trial process.
- Provide practical tips for delivering customer service to customers (study subjects) of clinical research studies.

Introduction

Customers continue to be the most valuable assets any organization can have. In the business of government, customers are *constituents*. In the hospitality industry they are guests. In clinical research we refer to clinical trial participants as *human subjects*, *volunteers* or *patients*. Regardless of what we call them, they are *customers*, and they keep the clinical research industry in business. Development of new compounds and therapies depends on clinical trial participants, and treating them as valued customers can have a dramatic impact on the successful outcome of patient recruitment, enrollment and retention efforts.

A business lesson learned the hard way from the recent high tech boom and bust is that the customer is now in charge.[1] That reality is also true for clinical research. Today's potential research study subjects are better educated, seek more healthcare information and assume more personal responsibility for health-related decisions than ever before. Their overall standards for service are also higher, and as a consequence the clinical research industry must offer quality customer service that matches the elevated expectations of these more informed and often demanding customers. This is especially true at a time when enrollment shortfalls and dropout rates for study subjects are at all-time highs.[2]

In order to reverse the current patient enrollment and retention trends, sponsors and investigative sites must act quickly and with resolve to create a culture of customer service, and develop new approaches to delivering quality service in every aspect of a clinical research study. A customer-centered culture requires customer-friendly policies, and barriers to service must be identified and eliminated.[3] How quickly and thoroughly these organizations integrate changes into service performance will be the measure of their success. There's a lot at stake, but also much to look forward to. A customer service strategy focused on delivering "meaningful and memorable" service has become a necessity. Meaningful change is not easy, but it is attainable, and the rewards will certainly justify the efforts required.

Commitment, Communication, Education and Leadership

Achieving meaningful changes in customer service requires commitment, communication, education and leadership.[4] It must be top-down and bottom-up, with participation throughout the organization in a team approach. It calls for a cultural commitment involving everyone in the organization. No one is exempt from the process. At the sponsor level it includes everyone from the CEO, President, Director of Clinical Research, to the Receptionist and Security Officer who welcome visitors to the facility. At investigative sites, it includes the principal investigator, study coordinator(s) and every staff member who interacts with candidates and enrolled study participants.

A superior customer service program begins with a commitment from upper management, and communication of the high-level goals and objectives throughout the organization.[5] Ideally, this is expressed as a mission statement, which defines the program's vision, purpose and objectives. Regardless of the form, it should be clear, concise, and reflect the commitment and values of the organization in its support of society and every patient participating in clinical research studies.

These values and objectives must then be adapted at various levels in order to reflect the specific needs and priorities of their particular customers. Only when senior management makes superior customer service a priority, will the rest of the organization take it seriously. And only when it is communicated all the way to the front lines will it be truly integrated into the attitudes and work habits of every employee.

Sample Mission Statement

Serving the best interests of society is our number one priority. We will strive to deliver superior customer service in all our dealings. We will treat everyone with friendliness, dignity and respect and work together as a team to develop strong relationships with our colleagues and customers.

Managers need to motivate, coach and empower their team members. They must find creative ways to spread the message. They must lead by example and raise their own service standards. Managers who find ways to make their people feel special will be surprised in ways they could not have predicted. To reinforce the principals of customer service, managers must acknowledge and reward actions that support a customer-centered culture. This can be accomplished by identifying daily opportunities for delivering service to individual staff members (internal customers), beginning with friendly greetings, positive feedback, encouragement, appreciation and recognition for their contributions in serving the team's efforts, or in achieving team goals. People will respond positively when it becomes personal for them, when they see and feel what it's like to be treated as a valued customer. Everyone needs to be part of customer service in action.

Staff members also need to participate in continuing education programs in order to deliver superior customer service. Customer service workshops, seminars and other in-service learning opportunities can be extremely valuable. Better-trained staff, with improved customer skills, will be more effective and project a more professional image. As they become more involved in processes that affect quality and continuous improvement, these people will gain an appreciation for the difference that each person can make. The effects of this approach can have powerful and lasting consequences for the entire organization. Relationships between Sponsors and investigative sites will improve, and the metrics gathered on patient enrollment and retention will reinforce the merits of these initiatives.

Defining Customer Service

Everyone in the organization (sponsor or site) must understand what it takes to deliver good customer service. They must recognize that customer needs, wants and expectations change, and the improvement process is ongoing and continuous. When this way of thinking permeates an organization, people begin to anticipate changing customer needs and wants, and they create solutions that can truly delight customers in meaningful and memorable ways.

What is good customer service? Simply put, it's about making the customer the number one priority—finding customer-friendly ways to deliver quality in every aspect of the way service is provided.[6] Service is all about people. It includes the people who work for sponsors, investigative sites (internal customers), and all those individuals who avail themselves of the products or services offered by those organizations (external customers), especially the patients involved in clinical research studies. Good customer service begins with identifying and acknowledging the need to satisfy fundamental human needs that are inherent in both internal and external customers, including the need to be listened to, appreciated, respected, trusted and valued. Within departments, standards should be determined in accordance with specific organizational needs, and those standards, in turn, must be aligned with how they can best satisfy all customers.

Making Service "Meaningful and Memorable"[7]

Raising the bar on customer service is not easy, but it is fundamentally simple. It's about improving customer relationships, with a focus on the little things that make big differences. Those little things can be defined as the ABC's of customer relationships—the Attitudes, Behaviors and Connections we have with customers.

- Attitudes—the way we feel about customers.
- Behaviors—the ways we act with customers.
- Connections—the ways we get involved with customers.

Suggestions for making the patient experience meaningful and memorable are offered in five service principals that can make the difference between success and failure for a clinical research study.

Service Principle 1

Know Thy Customer

To deliver superior customer service you must understand and be ready to satisfy your customers' needs, wants and expectations. Find out what matters most to your customers, and then demonstrate your service skills by what you actually do for them. By consistently demonstrating to your customers (study subjects), your knowledge and understanding of how they want to be treated, you help establish the foundation for a lasting relationship that is vital for the successful completion of a clinical research study. You will discover that a little investment in politeness, respect, patience, empathy and appreciation can return big dividends for your study.

A good service provider asks good questions and listens carefully to what customers say. Use a customer's name whenever possible, and as often as you can. Our name identifies us, makes us unique, and makes us feel special. Everyone who volunteers for a clinical trial is a very special person. Remembering to use a patient's name acknowledges, in a simple and personal way, that you appreciate them as individuals and value their continued participation in your study. It also expresses friendliness, a significant quality that resonates loudly with everyone. Remember that we are all customers.

Service Principle 2

Attitude Is Everything

Attitude can be defined as our emotional response to people, places, events and ideas and is expressed in our appearance, facial expression, body language, tone of voice and the words we choose to use. Attitudes leave impressions and impressions last. These mental impressions that will be recalled when potential study participants talk with their friends, relatives or caregivers about the attitudes expressed by the people they met or talked with while seeking more information about a clinical research study. Attitudes also determine people's actions, such as whether to show up for a screening appointment, whether to sign an Informed Consent Agreement, or whether to continue participation in a trial to its scheduled completion.

Attitudes can be classified into two basic categories; those that are healthy and those that are deadly. Healthy attitudes connect people. They are attractive, positive and productive. They are expressed in a friendly greeting, a warm smile, patient listening and a sincere, "Thank you." Deadly attitudes disconnect people. They are ugly and destructive and are demonstrated by frowns, smirks, unkind gestures, arguing or, deadliest of all, ignoring customers. Attitudes are easily detected, even in a telephone conversation, voice message, email or other forms of communication. And since attitudes are contagious, it is important to work at spreading the healthy ones, those that are worth catching. Here are some healthy and deadly attitudes.

Healthy Attitudes	Deadly Attitudes
I like you	I'm not interested in you
I respect you	I'm more important than you
I care about you	I'm too busy for you
I appreciate you	I'm right; you're wrong

The words we use, and how we use them, express and transmit our attitudes to colleagues and customers. And just as there are healthy attitudes and deadly attitudes, there are words to use (they connect us with customers) and words to lose (they disconnect us from customers).

Healthy Attitudes	Deadly Attitudes
Yes	I'm too busy
Certainly	You'll have to come back
Of course	That's not my job
I'd be happy to	You'll have to wait

Two of the most powerful and effective words you can ever use are "Thank you." Use them often, in face-to-face discussions, telephone conversations, and email messages. They tell people you care, you respect them and you appreciate them. They go a long way to alleviating anxiety and apprehension, establishing customer confidence and building the trusting relationship vital to a participant's enrolling in, and completing a clinical trial. Every customer contact offers opportunities to use "thank you" in a variety of situations. When a person calls to inquire about a study, that's an ideal opportunity to say, "Thank you for calling," or "Thank you for inquiring." When a question is asked, try saying "Thank you for asking," before giving the answer, and when someone shows up for a screening, that's a great opportunity to say "Thank you for coming in today," or "Thank you for keeping your appointment." When a customer has a complaint or problem, it's an opportunity to say "Thank you for bringing that to my attention." And when someone retrieves a telephone call that has been placed on hold, it's a great opportunity for that person to say, "Thank you for waiting." Most of all, when a customer signs an Informed Consent Agreement that's an ideal time to say "Thank you for agreeing to participate in this important study."

Just as a professional baseball player can improve his batting average every time he steps up to bat, everyone working on a clinical trial can improve their service performance by taking advantage of each "thank you" opportunity that presents itself. Customers feel special every time they hear those two special words, and when they respond with "You're welcome," a valuable customer connection has been made. The cumulative effect of each thank you is to build connections that help solidify the relationship, and develop the customer loyalty so necessary for patient retention, compliance and study completion.

Service Principle 3

Every Contact Counts

Every customer contact is a new opportunity for a meaningful connection and a chance to make a valuable deposit into a clinical trial's Customer

Relationship Account—one that can greatly appreciate in value over the time of a study's duration. As Steven Covey puts it, "In relationships, the little things are the big things."[8] Below are some typical opportunities for adding value to a study's customer relationship account. They may appear in personal contacts, emails, phone conversations, etc.

- The opportunity to learn more about your customer
- The opportunity to reinforce your customer's trust
- The opportunity to build customer loyalty
- The opportunity to ensure customer compliance and retention

Every one counts; they all add up, and they strengthen the customer relationship.

Service Principle 4

Keep It Simple and Sensible

People naturally resist anything complicated or confusing. Acceptance comes with clarity and understanding. Therefore, it is important for everyone involved in a clinical trial to have a clear and complete understanding of policies, procedures and regulations, and also be able to communicate them in terms that are easily understood. Applications, questionnaires, HIPAA forms and Informed Consent Agreements should be readable and make sense to the people who will be asked to sign them. Confusion, uncertainty, lack of clear understanding could result in a qualified candidate changing his or her mind about volunteering for a clinical research project. That would be a costly, yet avoidable loss.

One simple, sensible, yet often overlooked concept is remembering to smile. A smile costs nothing and is a valuable gift we can give customers every time we interact with them. A sincere smile speaks to customers in a universal language that says you care about them, you're interested in them, and you are connected to them in a positive way. It typically results in the recipient offering the gift of a smile in return. In addition, a smile has the power to break down barriers of fear and resistance and can be effortlessly transmitted over the telephone.

Service Principle 5

Practice Makes Permanent

We've all heard the phrase "practice makes perfect." Since we are all people and not one of us is ever perfect, expectations of achieving perfection are generally unrealistic. However, through practice, we can improve our customer service skills so they become permanent elements of our customer interactions, helping us to reinforce attitudes and actions that build customer relationships. Practice takes commitment, time, dedication and patience. It is repetitious and can be boring, but it is the most significant factor that separates amateurs from professionals, ordinary from exceptional. Practice produces habits of performance that delight customers, and it is delighted customers who become loyal customers. Whenever a friendly greeting, a warm smile or a sincere thank you becomes a habit that is delivered consistently, a high standard of service performance will be clearly achieved and conveyed. Habits are hard to change, both the good ones and the bad ones, and the customer habit that matters most in a clinical trial is the subject's habit of coming back to complete the study.

Creating Customer Magic

Everyone likes magic, and one thing that makes magic so memorable is the element of surprise, something unexpected. Making **A** Good Impression Count is **Customer MAGIC.**[9]

A clinical trial provides many opportunities for practicing Customer MAGIC. Whenever we do something surprising for a customer we go a long way to delighting them and reinforcing their decision to participate in a clinical trial. Making a good first impression in the initial customer contact is vital. However, every customer contact, whether it be a phone call, a screening visit or a follow-up meeting, sets the stage for making up to three good impressions. The first impression can be made in the way we connect with the customer—in our tone of voice, our friendly smile or a friendly greeting. The second impression can be made in how we *contribute* to our customer—how we answer a question or solve a problem—what we actually do for that person. A third good impression can be made in the way we *conclude* the interaction—whether we ask if there is anything else we can do for them, whether we thank them (for calling, for asking, etc.) and whether we extend to them a wish for a pleasant day. Thinking of creative ways to make good impressions and hopefully surprise customers can be challenging and rewarding. Whether the surprise comes from an unexpected smile, a sincere thank you, or simply the wish for a wonderful weekend, it will probably be the result of something simple and personal that makes it meaningful and memorable.

How Customers Evaluate Service

What are the standards people have for determining good service? Researchers have identified five customer-driven performance criteria, which create the acronym, **RATER.**[10]

Meaningful and Memorable Customer Service can be delivered when attitudes and actions demonstrate sensitivity and adherence to these criteria.

How Customers Evaluate Service

Reliability: accuracy, consistency, dependability
Assurance: knowledge, trust, competence, confidence
Tangibles: physical appearance of people and the workplace
Empathy: caring, attention, understanding
Responsiveness: timeliness and willingness to help

Summary

Raising the bar on customer service offers a challenging and achievable objective for the business of clinical research. It will take commitment, creativity and consistent effort on the part of everyone who works within sponsor and investigative site organizations. With clarity of purpose, patience, dedication and persistence, we can look forward to a clinical research industry that offers fewer delays and faster development cycles for promising new and treatments and therapies.

Key Takeaways

- A customer service culture must be adopted by the clinical research industry
- Volunteers for clinical research studies must be treated as valued customers
- Customer service training must be provided to everyone who interacts with participants throughout the cycle of a clinical research study
- Treating clinical trial participants as valued customers can have a direct impact on the success of patient recruitment and retention programs.
- Everyone involved with clinical research studies can make a contribution to raising the standards for customer service in clinical trials

References

1. *BusinessWeek*, "The Future of Tech/Road Map" August 25, 2003, Interview w/Sam Palmsano, IBM, p. 111.

2. "Improving Recruitment and Retention Practices Based on Input from the Public & Patients," CenterWatch, 2003.
3. Whiteley, Richard C., *The Customer-Driven Company*, The Forum Corp., 1991, Ch. 5, "Smash the Barriers to Customer-Winning Performance."
4. Leadership Ladder, Interview with Barbara Kenyon.
5. Ibid., *The Customer-Driven Company*, Ch.7, "Walk the Talk."
6. C. Leslie Charles, *Rule #1, Customer Service Handbook*, Successories Library, 1997, p. 9.
7. Think & Do, Improving Customer Relationships workshop topic, Copyright 1999.
8. Covey, Stephen R., *The Seven Habits of Highly Effective People*, Simon & Schuster, 1989, p. 192.
9. Ibid., Think & Do Workshops.
10. Dr. Leonard Barry, Texas A&M Researcher.

Author Biography

Steve Wishnack, B.A., M.S.
Founder, Think & Do™

Steve Wishnack is the founder and owner of Think & Do™, a company that delivers customer service workshops for improving customer relationships. www.thinkanddoworkshops.com

Steve holds both Bachelors and Masters degrees in Education from Brooklyn College, Brooklyn, NY. For the past thirty years' education, training and business development have been at the heart of Steve's professional career.

Today, Steve's energies are focused on providing consultation services, and on delivering his Think & Do Customer Service Workshops, which help improve individual effectiveness with customers and build customer loyalty. These hands-on, interactive programs have been successfully delivered to clients in both the public and private sectors, including High Tech, Banking and Finance, Hospitality, Tourism, and Health care. Among Steve's clients are the U.S. Postal Service, Hewlett-Packard, The Marriott Corporation, The Massachusetts Lodging Association, New York State Hotel & Tourism Association, as well as numerous Municipalities and Public Libraries.

For the past three years Steve has been involved with the Drug information Association (DIA) and has spoken on the topic of Customer Service at it's annual Patient Recruitment Conference. He has also been invited by Sponsors to talk about Customer Service at Investigator meetings and has been a guest speaker for the International Customer Service Association (ICSA).

13

Special Populations: Issues in the Recruitment of Women, Children and Minorities

Molly Mahoney Matthews, President and CEO, Matthews Media Group, Inc.
Leonard Sherp, Vice President, Matthews Media Group, Inc.

Objectives

- Gain understanding on reasons why women, members of multicultural communities and children are underrepresented as volunteers in clinical trials.
- Provide practical suggestions and proven outreach approaches to increase the participation of women, members of multicultural communities and children in clinical trials.

Introduction

Prescription medications treat, prevent and alleviate the symptoms of disease in people of all ages and ethnic backgrounds. The 85-year-old Hispanic grandmother, the young Caucasian father of three, the middle-aged African-American banker, the teenager, the child, Native Americans, Asian Americans—all these people may need medication at some point in their lives. Though medicines are prescribed to an incredibly diverse spectrum of Americans, clinical trials to assess their safety and effectiveness may not reflect this diversity.

Improving clinical trials participation rates among minorities, women and children is crucial to advancing the quality of healthcare for all people in the United States Though minority groups account for approximately a quarter of the U.S. population, only about five percent of participants in clinical trials are minorities.[1] Females were historically excluded from clinical trials because scientists believed hormonal fluctuations due to menstrual cycles would confound study data.[2] And only 20 to 30% of drugs approved by the U.S. Food and Drug Administration (FDA) are currently labeled for use in children.[3] This is a problem because people of different genders, ethnicities and age groups may metabolize medications differently.

For these reasons, special populations (defined for the purposes of this chapter as any group other than adult white males) have become a priority focus of clinical research over the past decade. Dating back to the years just after World War II, clinical testing was performed almost exclusively on adult white males, without much consideration as to whether this was good clinical practice or good policy. This began to change in the 1970s, albeit slowly and in fits and starts. Researchers started noticing that women and members of different ethnic and age groups often reacted differently to drugs than did the adult white males on whom these medications had been tested. By the early 1990s, the federal government got behind a movement to include women, minorities, children and adolescents in the pool of potential participants.

Regulatory Changes Mandate Including Special Populations in Clinical Research

This federal backing occurred in the form of sweeping policy change, which began by opening doors for women and minorities to participate in clinical research, and ultimately supported pediatric studies of certain medications. The National Institutes of Health (NIH) Revitalization Act of 1993 mandated that researchers include women and members of racial and ethnic minority groups in all federally funded, population-based studies. The following year, FDA lifted its ban on including women of childbearing age from early (phase I and early phase II) clinical studies. (This prohibition had been in place since 1977.) Four years later, in 1997, the federal government began opening regulatory doors to clinical research in pediatric populations.

The Food and Drug Modernization Act of 1997 (FDAMA) offered pharmaceutical companies financial incentives to conduct pediatric clinical trials for adult-approved medications that were already being widely prescribed to children and adolescents. The six-month exclusivity provisions of the 1997 FDAMA Act were extended in 2001, with passage of the Best Pharmaceuticals for Children Act (BPCA).[4] At the same time, legislation (The Pediatric Rule) was proposed to require pharmaceutical manufacturers to include pediatric data in any new drug submission for conditions that affect young people as well as adults (such as diabetes, hypertension, or obesity).[5]

On the heels of those initiatives, FDA issued the "Final Rule on Investigational New Drug Applications and New Drug Applications" (The Demographic Rule).[6] This 1998 regulation requires effectiveness and safety data for demographic subgroups (including gender, age and race) to be included in new drug applications (NDAs). It also mandates that investigational new drug application (IND) annual reports for drug and biological products include enrollment data for clinical studies subjects, tabulated by important demographic subgroups.

Socioeconomic, Cultural and Historical Factors Affect Recruitment Efforts

Mandating that special populations be included in clinical trials was one thing, but modifying study design and recruitment strategies to accomplish this goal proved no easy task. Social inequities that disproportionately affect minority populations (such as inadequate access to health insurance or quality health care[7]) combined with distrust of government institutions, posed serious barriers to minority recruitment. This was particularly true of African Americans, who harbor cultural memory of the shameful Tuskegee syphilis studies. These issues, combined with a paucity of minority investigators or culturally tailored recruitment strategies, continue to limit the number of people of color who volunteer for clinical trials.

The issue of pediatric involvement in clinical research is one that remains highly controversial. Intense media coverage of negative clinical research events may limit the pool of available participants. Despite these challenges, there have been many promising developments in special populations recruitment. Institutions and companies involved in clinical research have recognized the need to gain the public's trust and have begun the slow process of educating and reaching out to communities across America. NIH and FDA regulations for including women in clinical research have had an impact.[8] The BCPA confirmed the federal government's commitment to pediatric trials as the best means of ensuring that the medications we give our children are going to help—not harm—them. Pharmaceutical manufacturers have taken to heart FDA's appeals to represent the demographic profile of the U.S. population in clinical trials and have begun requiring defined age, gender and/or ethnic group cohorts in their protocols.

The promise of genomic medicine may lead us to medical therapies that are uniquely targeted to smaller groups of individuals. This and other new developments in medical research will make special populations outreach an increasingly vital component of successful drug development. Fortunately, our experiences over the past decade have taught us a great deal about how to recruit special populations. Communications strategies must honor the unique needs of people with different age, disability, ethnicity, gender, race and sexual identity backgrounds. Creative, effective recruitment strategies are critical to reaching groups traditionally underrepresented in clinical research. The following discussion explores some lessons learned and evolving best practices for ensuring those strategies are successful.

Recruitment of Women and Minorities

FDA's encouragement of the inclusion of women and minorities in clinical trials mirrors the changing demographics in the United States. Women have outnumbered men in the American population for decades, and by 2010, minority ethnic and racial groups will account for 32% of the population, up from 20% in 1980.[9]

This explosive growth in the number of non-white Americans has made it imperative that clinical trials include members of minority groups, not only because it is clinically and ethically prudent, but because it makes financial sense as well. Having representative numbers of minority group members as participants in clinical trials from their inception helps keep a drug's approval process on track and prevents having to backtrack and increase the research cohort size—and ethnic makeup—when the FDA orders a trial sponsor to do so. This is particularly true of drugs for health conditions that affect minority populations at a high rate. More recently, sponsors have found that in some cases, it makes sense to run additional studies exclusively for a minority group if such a group is affected disproportionately by a certain disease or treatment. Carefully designing inclusion criteria for clinical trials will help sponsors to swiftly take drugs from the lab to the marketplace without unnecessary delays.

Understanding the Need

Despite the push for inclusion, minority participation in clinical trials is vastly disproportional to these groups' representation within the public at large. FDA reports that racial and ethnic groups participate in clinical trials to varying degrees. There was a steady decline in participation by African Americans from 12% in 1995 to 6% in 1999. FDA estimates that this rate of participation by African Americans is representative of the U.S. population. However, at 3%, Hispanics appear to be underrepresented. Asians, Pacific Islanders and Native Hawaiians accounted for another 3%. Less than 1% were American Indians and Alaskan Natives.[10] More detailed information can be expected as the FDA continues to require Sponsors to comply with the reporting requirements of the 1998 Demographic Rule. According to CenterWatch, FDA medical reviewers have been given guidelines to increase their focus on minority inclusion.

The pharmaceutical industry must make an investment to get to know these special populations. As health communications firms have learned, clinical trial recruitment in diverse communities requires a combination of awareness, outreach and building trust.

Tuskegee: Today's Tragedy

The tragedy of the Tuskegee study continues to serve as a reminder to minority communities: (1) of the potential harm that can occur when clinical research is conducted without guidelines for participants' protection; and (2) of the disregard people of color have encountered from the medical and research community in the past. Although the Tuskegee study was by no means a clinical trial by today's standards, nonetheless it was a medical study, which is the message that the average citizen still hears and understands today.

To a layperson, the Tuskegee study design may look much like those of today. First, there is a terrible disease; second, researchers are looking for a treatment; third, people are recruited to take part in the research study; and fourth, some are given active treatment (study medication), while others might receive placebo in exchange for participation in the study and free medical exams. On the surface, this thumbnail sketch resembles the public's perception of today's clinical research, but, in fact, current procedural standards are quite different. How do we make those differences known?

As a first step in recruiting women and minorities to clinical trials, the Tuskegee study must be addressed honestly. We must educate the audience about current clinical trial procedures and how studies are designed. Efforts should be made to help potential study participants understand the value of the informed consent process and exactly what "informed consent" means (i.e., the rights of study volunteers to know the risks, potential benefits and other details of the study). Potential participants should also know what institutional review boards (IRBs) are and what function IRBs serve in protecting the integrity of the science and providing ethical constraints on study sponsors and investigators.

Until rigorous strides are made to help individuals from multicultural communities understand the clinical trial process and safety procedures that are in place today, a lack of understanding will continue to persist, along with a fear of participation in clinical trials. As a result, Tuskegee was recognized as a tragedy then—and still is today. Research efforts to advance the health and well-being of all people will continue to be hampered by this tragedy, to some extent, for years to come.

Special Populations Recruitment: Barrier or Challenge?

There is much talk about "barriers" to the recruitment of special populations into clinical trials. But to successfully enroll these hard-to-reach groups, we should view barriers not as insurmountable obstacles but as discrete challenges that can be addressed and overcome, one at a time, with careful, targeted programs, as the examples that follow suggest.

Barrier: Mistrust

The first barrier is the fear and mistrust, stemming from the Tuskegee legacy.

Addressing the Challenge of Mistrust

Information on the clinical trial process must be made readily available in the community of the intended audience and delivered by messengers and vehicles they trust. That may require community-based health workers or others trained in the clinical trial process to be available as clinical trial educators to offer information and answer questions on what to expect in a clinical trial. Recruitment materials are often generated for specific trials, but sponsors might want to include culturally sensitive informational pieces on the clinical trials process in general.

Barrier: "I Won't Be Your Guinea Pig"

People sometimes view research as an opportunity for a sponsor to enter a community, perform research or "tests" on human subjects and leave without contributing to the needs and concerns of the community.

Addressing the "Guinea Pig" Challenge

At the start of any particular study, sponsors should plan to leave behind a contribution to the community. Small efforts, such as the development of a scholarship program to assist others in becoming researchers, or equipment such as blood pressure cuffs and monitors in community centers, go a long way in generating a positive and lasting impression.

Barrier: "I've Got Bigger Problems"

Women and minorities who decline to participate in clinical trials often say they have more immediate and bigger problems to address than their own health concerns or the prevention of a disease they currently don't have or may never get.

Addressing the "Bigger Problems" Challenge

Many studies suggest people join clinical trials not only because they hope to improve a health problem, but also because they believe they can make a contribution to society. Tapping into that sense of volunteerism can be effective in some communities, at least as a strategy to generate interest in asking more about a trial. This should be addressed through an effective recruitment plan that weaves together disease-specific information, awareness-raising activities, study-related information and a sense of altruism.

Barrier: "But I Have No Health Insurance"

Many underserved populations avoid contact with the medical system because they have no way to pay for their care. According to the United States Census Bureau, in 2001, 33% of Hispanics, 19% of African Americans, 18% of Asian and Pacific Islanders, and 10% of Caucasians did not have health insurance.[11] Researchers who ask patients to rely on health insurance for continued care at the conclusion of the study will be excluding a large percentage of potential enrollees.

Addressing the "No Health Insurance" Challenge
Studies that do not require health insurance and are administered at no cost to participants will likely be the most effective. That message, however, must be clearly conveyed.

Barrier: "I Don't Want Others to Know My Medical History"
Many people are afraid to share their medical history for fear that their information will become part of a larger "data bank." The underlying fear is that potential employers will somehow receive this information and use it as a means to deny employment.

Addressing the "Medical History" Challenge
The recently updated Health Insurance Portability and Accountability Act (HIPAA)[12] offers a new layer of privacy for study subjects. However, it is, at best, a complicated law to understand. It is not enough for sponsors to hand out a series of complicated forms for the potential enrollee to sign. Sponsors should also consider adding an easy-to-read publication that explains HIPAA protections.

Barrier: "It's Not in My Neighborhood"
Transportation is often listed as a barrier to participation in clinical trials. Participants aren't likely to travel more than 25 miles for a study.

Addressing the "It's Not in My Neighborhood" Challenge
Research should be conducted to identify the communities with a high morbidity rate for the disease being studied. The smart sponsor then considers incorporating sites located in inner city, urban and rural locations to attract particular audiences. As a benefit, locating a site in the neighborhood of intended audiences links the trial with a particular health center or physician and stands a good chance of becoming a well-known study throughout the community.

Barrier: "But He's Not My Doctor"
Minorities who are in the healthcare system prefer the clinician they know and trust. Currently, only 6% of U.S. physicians are minorities (African American, Native American or Hispanic)[13] and very few participate in research. For many minority patients, their primary care doctor is their most valuable and trusted source of health information.

Addressing the "Not My Doctor" Challenge
There are few programs in place to encourage minority physicians to participate in research. Study sponsors would be wise to promote programs that

break down the level of disinterest and distrust that exists among minority clinicians. Minority investigators would help attract the populations that sponsors are seeking.

Efforts to include as many minority investigators and study coordinators as possible should also be considered. In doing so, research and procedural training for new investigators and study coordinators might be necessary. The cost of exposing new investigators to the study process may seem excessive, but once educated about the process, they will be much better prepared for the next study.

Barrier: "I Can't Leave Work"

The typical 8:30 to 5:00 doctor's appointment hours may not accommodate working people's schedules. To the extent that minority group members are more often economically disadvantaged and occupying jobs with less flexible attendance schedules—or leave benefits—"normal" doctors' hours limit their participation in clinical trials.

Addressing the "Can't Leave Work" Challenge and Allowing for Flexibility

Studies that offer site and call center hours beyond the traditional 8:30 to 5:00 period can markedly increase participation, especially among candidates with no medical or personal leave to spare. Many sites now opt to offer appointment visits during extended office hours at least one or two days a week.

Barrier: What if the Drug Is not Available at the Conclusion of the Study?

For many, continued treatment at the conclusion of a study is of particular concern. Many who received the study drug and experienced considerable benefits might be told they can no longer have access to the medication. This is definitely a disincentive to participation.

Addressing the "Conclusion of the Study" Challenge

Unblinding the drug at the study's end and offering an open label extension may serve as one option to counter this reaction; however, it is often not part of the protocol design. In that case, participants must be made aware at the time of study consent that upon conclusion of the study, the drug will not be available for continued use. If, on the other hand, the study's design allows for continued use due to it involving research of an already FDA-approved drug, Sponsors should make efforts to verify the participant's coverage of the study drug or inform participants of alternatives (e.g., programs that supply the drug at reduced or no cost) should they not have health insurance. In the long run, pharmaceutical Sponsors may want to consider offering lifelong access to medication at no charge for participants in clinical trials that contributed to that drug's approval.

Out-of-the-Box and In-Your-Community Recruitment Strategies

In developing outreach strategies to reach special populations, sponsors must be willing to enter communities and work to enlist their support. While national outreach and advertising are useful, local outreach helps to build trust among wary populations.

Ambassador Program

MMG has developed an innovative outreach program, enlisting community members as "ambassadors" to take a grassroots approach to reach the target study populations and educate them about the study. As frontline campaign representatives, ambassadors assist in gathering valuable information about the target population that is then used to develop a more successful and progressive recruitment strategy. Ambassadors come from all walks of life. They can be college students, teachers, clergy or anyone with the trust of the community. The most effective ambassadors are quite familiar with the target population and have built-in access to their gathering spots. When ambassadors are accepted in the community as trustworthy and knowledgeable, they can effectively gather information about the needs of the target audience and help explain and publicize the study. The ambassador program has proven to be a highly effective tool for the recruitment of special populations when coupled with other recruitment strategies.

Advocacy Groups as Partners

Development of organizational partners, who agree to lend their support on behalf of a particular study—especially those organizations with grassroots reach—has also proven to be an effective recruitment tool. Potential participants are more open to joining a clinical trial when it is presented to them by an organization to which they already belong or trust. Not only does this build credibility and trust for the study, it also allows Sponsors to reach large numbers of potential participants through cost-effective means. National associations and organizations, local libraries and hospitals, and even local churches can be considered as prospective partners. However, study Sponsors must be open to sharing the study design and protocol with organizational partners in order to garner their support.

Pediatric Recruitment

For pharmaceutical companies, pediatric trials offer the means to expand a medication's approved indications, bringing valuable therapies to a needy population while simultaneously protecting and enhancing formidable opportunities in an increasingly competitive marketplace.

Children themselves carry widely different perspectives about clinical research participation. Being a patient in a trial can create a sense of pride for one young person who values the distinction of being selected to support research that will benefit many others with the same illness. To another child in that same study, trial participation is not a badge of honor but a burden—reminder and further reinforcement that children with illnesses are different.

With the many other competing or conflicting issues involved—flavored by a mix of individuals and organizations whose goals and concerns are frequently at odds—recruitment for pediatric clinical trials presents a unique set of challenges. Successful patient recruitment for pediatric trials demands a multifaceted understanding of the motivations and expectations of patients, parents, siblings, physicians and other healthcare providers, regulators, researchers and sponsors. Equally important, the clinical research team must possess both the skill and experience to communicate directly and effectively with each of these groups. As discussed throughout this chapter, these challenges are complicated by the fact that the current climate for medical research places premiums on accelerated recruitment, requiring rapid response to a study protocol's needs with little time for reflection.

Overlooked and Understudied

For years, medications prescribed for children for illnesses shared with adults (e.g., diabetes, asthma, bipolar disorder) were rarely tested specifically on a pediatric population, and dosage recommendations were simply weight-based recalculations of approved adult dosages. In many cases, doctors and parents simply mashed up adult doses into applesauce to make them palatable to and—it was hoped—safe and effective for their youngest patients. Such guesswork seemed to be the only response possible in the absence of clinically tested guidance on pediatric dosing.

The term "therapeutic orphans" historically has been used to describe the state of neglect that has befallen children in pharmaceutical research—a situation that extended well into the waning years of the twentieth century. But the legislative and regulatory thrusts described at the beginning of this discussion have changed all that. Therapeutic orphans no more, children and adolescents have now been thrust front and center into the world of clinical research. Those involved in that recruitment—sponsors, investigators and outsourcing agencies—have had to focus on the problems and particulars of finding, enrolling and maintaining patients in pediatric trials, some of which are described in the following points.

A Look at the Children

What criteria define a pediatric patient? The answer might seem obvious, but criteria and definition are basic to recruitment for pediatric clinical trials. Toddlers are definitely pediatric patients, but so too, according to FDA guidelines, are 16-year-olds. On the other hand, 17-year-olds may not be. The enormous disparities in physical development between a first grader and a teenager raise certain flags and will obviously affect study design. In selected pediatric studies that have broad age inclusion (i.e., ages 6 to16) and are being conducted under FDA guidelines, FDA has requested that sponsors make efforts to ensure that their study population be stratified by age and balanced by cohort. For example, a certain percentage of the study cohort must be grouped between ages 6 and 10, with an equal percentage aged 11 to 16. This stratification is intended to capture data on any differences in the drug's efficacy and utilization that occur across varying stages of physical development. Similarly, the developmental differences between girls and boys suggest, for certain compounds, the need to assure a representative sample of both sexes in the study. Requiring representative numbers of participants from different age groups and both genders in turn impacts recruitment strategies and methods.

Coupled with these factors are the even greater disparities in social development. Younger children are likely to listen to their parents and take medications when told; teenagers decidedly less so. Teenagers may have the ability to read and understand an informed consent document, but few elementary school-aged children can. Moreover, the soaring sense of self and power that accompanies adolescence may make teenagers unwilling even to admit they are ill. To do so, and to further acknowledge illness by participating in a clinical trial, amounts to an acceptance of their own limitations, a dent in their belief in their own invincibility. That belief resonates with particular strength among certain ethnic teenagers, who place great emphasis on the virtues of strength and stoicism associated with adulthood.

For those attempting to recruit for pediatric trials, these social differences will affect the kinds of messages crafted and the media in which they appear. Who is the proper spokesperson, Big Bird or a cast member from *Dawson's Creek* or *The Osbournes*? What's a better retention item, a CD carrying case or a coloring book? Is advertising placed on radio stations that attract teen listeners, or should it focus only on the stations that appeal to their parents, who in the end will have to make the ultimate decision about their child's participation?

Our experience has revealed techniques and approaches that address the variations in recruiting for pediatric clinical trials. For young people who have already expressed pride in volunteering and participating, recognition of their efforts can be as simple as a well-designed certificate of appreciation, or include a variety of retention items, such as hats, T-shirts or water bottles bearing a study's logo and name.

A comic book—which used a superhero-based narrative line to explain a study, its goals and the altruistic aspects of participation—proved to be a compelling, highly effective and "kid-friendly" communication tool. Extensive planning efforts were invested to assure that the comic book's language and underlying message were not coercive and presented a balanced view on trial participation, emphasizing the significance of language and choice in attracting young people to a research study. Just as the dramatic but tailored story line of a comic book proved to be a successful recruitment tool, a shopping mall screening table drew far more children (and parents) on behalf of a juvenile diabetes study with a banner asking "Does Diabetes Run in Your Family?" than would one simply stating "Free Diabetes Screening."

Altruism and community welfare are meaningful concepts to children, more than many adults realize. Young people take pride in highly developed social values, and advertising messages that invoke or reinforce these values are inevitably more successful than straightforward announcements of medical research efforts. The mainstream logic of public relations would hold that use of the word "free" is always the best attractor, but we learned that speaking to altruism was, in fact, a greater attractor. This observation underscores a pivotal concept in recruiting children to clinical trials: children and adolescents respond to advertising and calls to action that are not only communicative, succinct and easy to remember, but invoke a sense of family care, concern and social responsibility.

An example of these applied strategies is a recent recruitment campaign for a drug to treat depression in young children and adolescents. The pharmaceutical company client set the goal to recruit 265 children, ages 6 to 17, to a two-armed (one fixed dose, one flexible dose), placebo-controlled trial with more than 25 sites throughout the country over a 15-month period. Different advertising techniques were used in tougher areas (e.g., Los Angeles and Denver) and three television ads, pertaining to different aspects of the disorder, were used to encompass seasonal and age distribution fluctuations. The results: recruitment was completed on time with 285 total randomizations and with an even balance of child and adolescent participants in the trial.

Recruiting Children—And Their Parents

The key role parents must play in pediatric recruiting underscores the fact that recruitment among children focuses only partially on the child who may happen to have the specific medical condition that meets a drug protocol's inclusion criteria. After all, it is the parent or guardian who provides legal authorization for a child to participate in a clinical trial. It is the parent or guardian who will struggle with issues of benefit and risk. It is the parent or guardian, in addition to the child, with whom study coordinators and investigators will discuss the rights and responsibilities of a study subject, informed consent and the importance of placebo. It is therefore the entire family who are the communications target audience for clinical trials involving children.

But the role of a child's parent or guardian in a pediatric trial transcends the clinical and legal requirements for participation. When recruiting for pediatric clinical trials, especially studies that require newly or non-diagnosed patients or those not receiving medication, it is the parent's or guardian's antennae that must be reached. A child may not want to go to school or play with friends, but it is the parent or guardian who must first question whether these behaviors reflect an emotional or personality disorder. Parents face these quandaries all the time—for example, when can a teenager's problem with weight be reclassified as obesity? And, if so reclassified, how much medical attention is justified or appropriate? Should this child enter a weight-reduction or hypertension study, and, if so, how?

A similar line of questioning has surrounded the efficacy of the stimulant methylphenidate (Ritalin). At what point is an ebullient and energetic child, in fact, dysfunctionally hyperactive and in need of intervention? Are clinical screening instruments for hyperactivity and attention-deficit disorders accurate? What do we really know about the effects of amphetamine-based stimulants in children? This debate, with its swamp of troubling and unanswered questions, illustrates the ambiguity that exists for medical providers, researchers and parents when faced with making rational and humane decisions about what constitutes normal childhood behavior and what demands medical intervention.

In the course of navigating such difficult ethical terrain, the very act of acknowledging a child's illness or susceptibility to illness, the usual *sine qua non* of clinical research, may be viewed as an indictment of parenting ability. In the case of the obese child sought for a hypertension study, for example, many parents might be reluctant to admit their overweight children are in fact obese, an often pejorative label that could imply they did not provide proper nutrition or are unable to control their child's impulses. Recruiting children for trials involving mood disorders or mental illness raises similar challenges as parents wonder why they cannot ease their child's anxieties or fears, and at what level of severity these fears constitute a "diagnosis" that infers a parenting failure.

Equally important as familial attitudes toward illness are cultural perspectives exhibited by different ethnic groups. Shyness has recently been identified as a behavioral diagnosis and trials are already being designed to test certain drugs that may offer symptomatic relief. In families of Middle Eastern origin, where custom limits a child's exposure to social situations, extraordinary shyness—clinically diagnosable shyness—will go unrecognized. Similarly, in contrast to the American fascination with waif-like thinness as a mark of beauty, South Asian tradition places a premium on fullness. Recruitment for childhood obesity trials might fall on deaf ears in that population. Expressions of pain or discomfort are discouraged among many African American or Latino boys, in keeping with the general dictates of their cultures—a factor that could limit their willingness (or familial interest) in participating in studies investigating analgesics.

While some parents are reluctant to identify their children as potentially eligible candidates for clinical research for either cultural or attitudinal reasons, others find clinical trials to be a route to otherwise unavailable medical care for their children. A clinical trial may be the last and only avenue to the level of physician care that can offer true hope for impoverished children and families, and which bring access to specialist physicians denied to them under managed care or insurance-based programs.

Whatever the route that opens the way for a parental decision, be it economic need or overcoming philosophical or sociocultural objections, recognizing that a child might qualify for a clinical trial is only the first step that demands parental and familial involvement. Once a child is accepted into a study, compliance becomes a family activity. Someone has to accompany the child on every visit to the research study center, which may be located far from the neighborhood. A parent must take time away from work, brothers and sisters miss school, and in-laws may be called upon to help with transportation or stay with younger children at home during study visits. Medication must be taken on time, diets may have to change, study diaries need to be maintained—all of which have an impact on a family's regular activities. Invariably, the fact that every family has a unique set of interdependencies will one way or another be reflected in a child's enrollment and participation in a pediatric clinical trial.

Familial relationships also affect a child's participation in clinical research in other, subtler ways. If a child senses that the family deems it important to continue in a study, the child may experience (even if it is never overtly stated) a quiet pressure to remain uncomplaining. This, in turn, can lead a study participant to withhold information when not feeling well in order to not disappoint, or to hide or understate symptoms to avoid rebuke for not being a "good patient." The desire to accommodate expectations typically extends to the relationship a child develops with the research team as well. The possibility that a child may subvert his or her personal experience in order to please an adult authority figure, parent or otherwise, needs to be considered when crafting and explaining informed consent materials. This issue becomes even starker when monetary reimbursement is provided for participation. Imagine the pressure on a child from a family of little means whose honest answer to the questions; "Is everything okay?" or "Any problems since you started taking the new medicine?" could cost the family dollars.

Sites That Work

If the psychological and cultural issues impacting pediatric clinical trials are formidable, other equally difficult logistical concerns affect pediatric recruitment. The choice of principal investigator (PI), site location and amenities, and study support with communication and outreach tools might seem elementary, the ordinary nuts and bolts of running a study. Still, these points often escape those involved in structuring and executing recruitment for trials.

Sponsors of clinical research routinely look to an investigator's past and current patient panels as rich sources for trial patients. At times, the specific nature of a physician's practice, patient catchments and demographics, or the economic indicators driving medical care choices in the physician's area, are either superficially assessed or not included in an overall assessment of any given doctor's suitability as an Investigator. When recruiting for an unusual genetic disorder or pediatric cancer trials, signing pediatric specialists and sub-specialists as investigators would logically be the best route for research Sponsors, since children with these conditions are nearly always referred for specialty care.

On the other hand, pediatric rheumatologists may not be the most successful recruiters or investigators for a chronic fatigue study that seeks children as yet undiagnosed and untreated. Those patients are more likely to be identified initially by their primary care pediatricians or family practice teams, including physicians, physician assistants and nurse practitioners.

Office hours are another consideration. As noted previously, the standard 8:30 to 5:00 regimen doesn't lend itself to optimal participation for pediatric trials. During most of those hours, children are in school and many parents are reluctant to have them miss more class time than they normally would. It also means that working parents, who would have to accompany their children for the office visits required by the study, must miss work—a luxury many simply cannot afford. Solutions seem simple—later hours, weekend appointments—but too often researchers and their staffs are unwilling to revise schedules to accommodate their pediatric trial participants' needs.

Basic amenities at a research site matter to children and their parents or guardians. Waiting rooms should have play areas, children's books and art that appeal to pediatric patients. Such factors go a long way toward taking the sting out of a child's office visit by offering activities to occupy them during the often long or unexpected waits that may occur and helping to take their minds off what may be an uncomfortable and fearful experience.

Lessons Learned

Despite daunting challenges, recruitment for pediatric and adolescent clinical trials can succeed, provided that those involved in recruitment are aware of the challenges and take carefully planned steps to meet them. Based on our experiences in recruiting for pediatric clinical trials on behalf of both government and industry sponsors, a group of useful guidelines for pediatric recruitment initiatives have emerged that are both illustrative of recruiting needs and applicable across a variety of clinical research objectives.

Motivate Mothers

Promotional materials and advertising placements for pediatric trials need to target parents more than children. In most families this means mothers, since mothers usually make decisions about health care, especially a child's health. Advertising campaigns must target mothers' listening and reading habits. Because many mothers respond to concerns raised by other mothers, testimonial-based advertising is also quite effective.

When distributing materials, a corner beauty salon where women get their hair done is a better location for a poster seeking kids for an asthma study than the local video arcade where children with asthma may spend much of their free time. The "easy listening," oldies or soft rock stations that appeal to adult listeners are more appropriate for radio advertising than the hard rock and rap stations adolescents favor. Daytime television targeted to women (talk shows, *Oprah*, daytime dramas) offer sensible points for airing TV commercials in support of pediatric trials, as opposed to Saturday morning children's programming or *Monday Night Football*.

Motivate Children

The idea that a clinical trial may provide a remedy for a child's health-related problem could be a powerful incentive for a parent. It may not, on the other hand, be such a potent motivator for the child who must take a medication, give up Saturday mornings or have blood drawn on a regular basis. To offset the obvious misgivings a child might experience when faced with these options, an attempt must be made to instill a sense of uniqueness and significance in clinical trial participation. It works far better, from a young person's perspective, if a study is memorable in the way other child-focused products are: with bright color schemes, a memorable name (such as an easy acronym), a well-designed logo and individualized graphics.

Incentive items can underscore a study's recognition factor with participants, creating a further resonance with consistent and clearly designed graphic elements on study materials such as posters and brochures. One successful incentive example is a recognition program that tracks each visit and specifically thanks children for their efforts on behalf of a study. After each visit a child can redeem a visit recognition certificate for an appreciation item. Conveying uniqueness, offering a degree of pleasure and reward and underscoring a child's sense of pride in making a valued contribution are all methods of both "branding" a study and offering an opportunity to enhance and maximize communication between children and their parents, as well as among participating families, investigators, and site personnel.

Access Intermediary Groups

Parents rely on trusted individuals, organizations and institutions for information. These include advocacy groups, churches, their children's schools, their pediatricians and clinics. Outreach to these organizations, at both the local and national levels, can provide valuable allies in raising awareness among parents about their children's health and their options for treatment, including clinical trials. Specific advocacy- or intermediary-based outreach techniques that have proven successful in bringing patients to clinical trials include:

- Disease-specific screenings held at churches or in community clinics ("Does Diabetes Run in Your Family?")

- Informational seminars at churches, libraries or community centers that present, discuss and answer questions about a trial and its objectives
- Direct mailings from established advocacy groups on behalf of a trial, with contact points for more information
- Articles placed in advocacy newsletters or content on advocacy web sites about a clinical trial with contact points for more information about sites and screening criteria
- Partnerships between advocacy groups and research sites to share resources and optimize access by and for potential participants
- Promotional support for advocacy groups and sites with professionally created graphics and communications solutions

It's a Family Affair

Remembering that children cannot elect to enroll themselves in clinical trials is critical in the implementation of strategies aimed at successful and large-scale recruitment of children. Families must be the focus and target of virtually all marketing and communication outreach efforts, and various points of timing and placement become important in reaching children—and their parents. If random intercepts or off-site screenings are an important element in recruitment, choose sites and times when children will actually be accompanying their parents. Rather than schedule an event at a local mall for Saturday, when kids go there to be with their friends and to get away from their parents, think about a back-to-school sale day when the family is shopping together. Include the family when designing incentive packages and retention programs. A dinner for four, a trip to the movies, or a day at the ballpark are all ways to effectively say thanks for the efforts of children and their families on behalf of a trial. All too often, such participation and sacrifice go unrewarded by investigators and sponsors.

Pediatric Clinical Trials at a Crossroads

For the first time in the history of modern medicine and pharmaceutical development, regulatory and legislative mandates are fueling substantive research initiatives on behalf of children's health. Despite this growing national trend, the challenges remain significant, not the least of which involve complex ethical issues surrounding familial beliefs about health and medicine, children's understandable hesitancy about being research subjects, and the various institutional and industry needs to maximize recruiting goals.

For far too long, children shared with the elderly the problem of being at the nearly invisible edge of the social continuum: out of the way and off the economic chart. Yet the welfare of children lies at the heart of our strongest cultural and spiritual imperatives and, with that, holds a definitive social and scientific importance for all of us. Successful pediatric clinical trial recruitment demands vigorous, eclectic and innovative approaches to the array of issues, concerns, needs and individuals involved in the multi-tiered business of clinical trials. The vital thread that has proven consistently effective in linking strategies to children, parents and investigators rests in keeping all recruiting efforts participant-centered, as well as remembering the fundamental mission for all concerned: improving the health of children everywhere.

Summary

Over the past decade, the federal government has instituted a number of regulatory reforms encouraging researchers to recruit women, minorities, and children into clinical studies. These policies constitute an important first step towards accumulating data to assess the safety and effectiveness of medications for all appropriate population subgroups. Yet policy change alone is insufficient to ensure successful special populations recruitment efforts. Socioeconomic, cultural and historical factors affect potential participants' willingness and/or perceived ability to take part in clinical studies. In addition, negative media publicity about clinical research has led many members of the public to feel distrustful of clinical research. If they are uncomfortable with the idea of volunteering for a clinical trial themselves, they are likely to be even more nervous about enrolling their child. Researchers must address these obstacles to recruitment by reaching out to communities to address their concerns, and to educate them about the process of clinical research.

Tailored communication strategies that take into account the beliefs, attitudes and concerns of specific subpopulations are more likely to be effective. In recruiting special populations, researchers must take the time to understand how these audiences make decisions, and what factors influence their choices. This information helps develop culturally appropriate interventions that honor the concerns of their target audience. Efforts to recruit children must also bear in mind the specific age of the child, and the role of the parent in making decisions about that child's health care.

Customized outreach and communications ensure that women, minorities and children who may be eligible to participate in a clinical study receive the information they need to make this critical healthcare decision. The end result will be improved clinical trials participation rates and higher quality of care for all Americans.

Key Takeaways

- Greater participation of women, minority group members, children and adolescents in clinical trials is essential to ensure adequate data on the safety and efficacy of prescription medications among all the people for whom those medications may be prescribed.

- As is the case for all good patient recruitment efforts, when seeking to recruit among any of these special populations, put the potential patients' concerns first and design outreach programs to meet those concerns.
- Special populations recruitment requires special outreach programs. Think creatively.

References

1. Maxwell C, Goosby E, Mody V et al. Deadly Diseases and People of Color: Are Clinical Trials an Option? U.S. Food and Drug Administration, July 10, 1998. http://www.fda.gov/oashi/patrep/welcomeandopeningremarks.html
2. Killien M, Bigby J, Champion V et al. "Involving Minority and Underrepresented Women in Clinical Trials: The National Centers of Excellence in Women's Health." *Journal of Women's Health and Gender-based Medicine*, Vol. 9 (10), 2000.
3. Meadows M. "Drug Research and Children: Recent studies are providing important information about drug safety and effectiveness for children. Pediatricians say its about time." U.S. Food and Drug Administration, *FDA Consumer Magazine*, January-February, 2003. http://www.fda.gov/fdac/features/2003/103_drugs.html
4. U.S. Department of Health and Human Services, Food and Drug Administration, "Best Pharmaceuticals for Children Act." http://www.fda.gov/opacom/laws/pharmkids/contents.html
5. U.S. Department of Health and Human Services, Food and Drug Administration. "Regulations Requiring Manufacturers to Assess the Safety and Effectiveness of New Drugs and Biological Products in Pediatric Sites and Patients, Proposed Rule." 21CFR 201, 312, 314, 601. Federal Register. August 15, 1997. Vol. 62, p. 43900.
6. U.S. Department of Health and Human Services, Food and Drug Administration, "Investigational New Drug Applications and New Drug Applications, Final Rule." Federal Register. February 11, 1998; 63(8):6854-62.
7. *America Becoming: Racial Trends and Their Consequences*, eds. Neil J. Smelser, William Julius Wilson, and Faith Mitchell (Washington, D.C.: National Academy Press), Volume I, 530 pp.; Volume II, 492 pp. Volume I ISBN (hc): 0-309-06495-3; (pb): 0-309-06838-X. Volume II ISBN (hc) 0-309-06839-8; (pb): 0-309-06840-1.
9. Prout MN, Fish SS. "Participation of Women in Clinical Trials of Drug Therapies: A Context for The Controversies." *Medscape General Medicine* 3(4), 2001.

10. "Demographic Trends and the Burden of Disease." *Health & Health-care 2010, The Forecast, The Challenge, Institute for the Future.* Chapter 2, p. 19.

11. Evelyn B, Toigo T, Banks D, *Participation of Racial/Ethnic Groups in Clinical Trials and Race-Related Labeling: A Review of New Molecular Entities Approved 1995-1999.* U.S. Department of Health and Human Services, Food and Drug Administration. http://www.fda.gov/cder/reports/race_ethnicity/race_ethnicity_report.htm

12. Mills RJ. *Health Insurance, 2001.* U.S. Census Bureau, September, 2001. http://www.census.gov/prod/2002pubs/p60-220.pdf

13. Health Insurance Portability and Accountability Act (HIPAA), U.S. Public Law 104-191, August 4, 1996 http://aspe.hhs.gov/admnsimp/pl104191.htm

14. Institute for the Future, *Health and Health Care 2010: The Forecast, The Challenge*, Jossey-Bass Publishers, San Francisco, January, 2000.

Author Biographies

Molly Mahoney Matthews
Founder, President and CEO of Matthews Media Group, Inc. (MMG)

Molly Mahoney Matthews is the founder, president and chief executive officer of Matthews Media Group, Inc. (MMG), a strategic health communications firm in Rockville, Maryland. Ms. Matthews is a lifelong business leader and educator committed to improving health care for all Americans, particularly minority and historically underserved populations.

Ms. Matthews founded MMG in 1987. Her interest in clinical trial recruitment grew out of her early communications work with the National Institutes of Health (NIH). MMG is now a full-service healthcare, public relations and marketing firm, specializing in communications, clinical trial patient recruitment, social marketing and outreach to diverse populations. The company works in both the pharmaceutical and government sectors.

Under Ms. Matthews' leadership, MMG has developed a participant-centered focus in providing patient recruitment services to NIH and the pharmaceutical industry, a unique recruitment model that includes working closely with community-based clinics, partnering with intermediary organizations, and utilizing local and national media strategies.

In the year 2000, MMG was acquired by Diversified Agency Services (DAS) of Omnicom Group, Inc. Omnicom's DAS is a global organization offering services in direct marketing, consultancy, public relations, promotional marketing and specialty communications. DAS companies serve clients worldwide through 550 offices in more than 65 countries. Ms. Matthews continues to serve as MMG's president and CEO.

Ms. Matthews was selected for the Leadership Washington class of 2000. She is a member of the Board of Trustees at St. Mary's College of Maryland.

Leonard Sherp
Vice President of Matthews Media Group, Inc. (MMG)

A managing vice president at MMG, Leonard Sherp is a versatile communications professional with more than 30 years' experience in writing, media relations, community relations, event planning and project management for clients in the public and private sectors. During his 5-years at MMG, Mr. Sherp has directed a number of clinical trial recruitment programs (including pediatric trials) and played a lead role in developing new business opportunities with commercial clients.

Prior to joining MMG in 1998, Mr. Sherp managed the media relations and publications program for a major academic medical center and operated his own communications company, with clients ranging from an educational company developing new curricula for middle school children to a national presidential campaign. He has written or produced almost every conceivable kind of marketing material, print and electronic; organized award-winning media conferences; engineered medial placements for scores of clients; managed projects of national scope and outreach; and supervised staff of diverse talents and skills.

PART THREE

Case Studies

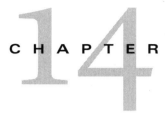

CHAPTER

The Investigative Site–Third-Party Provider Relationship

Pamela Kivitz-Keenan, Altoona Center for Clinical Research

Objectives
- Strategies for SMO and investigative sites communication and advertising coordination.
- Methods for:
  - Increasing study awareness.
  - Focusing advertising, even with national campaigns.
  - Personalizing the patient experience.

Introduction

The investigative site faces many challenges and competition when participating in today's clinical research studies. The site should be attentive to the recruitment process, ensuring a higher success rate of patient enrollment as well as in developing techniques for retention of patients. The demand for greater site involvement, more stringent inclusion/exclusion criteria and increased competition from other investigative sites has resulted in many new creative and innovative recruitment initiatives. It has become necessary for investigative sites to develop techniques for recruiting and retaining study patients in order to be recognized as effective and efficient.

Investigative sites vary greatly, from their actual physical size and staff volume, to their sophistication and ability to market effectively for different protocols. While some sites are not over-burdened with the prospect of initiating their own marketing campaign for a study, other sites lack the internal resources or expertise to work independently on a full marketing campaign.

In addition, third-party providers are increasingly popular and helpful in managing sponsor and site recruitment initiatives. Third party providers have become more alluring for a sponsor to use due to their centralized approach, information flow and level of expertise they can bring to numerous investigative sites. However, these providers can, at times, lack an in-depth understanding of local media markets and patient populations. Therefore, as both sides bring distinct assets to the relationship, it is imperative for the third-party providers and investigative sites to develop a partnership to maximize resources and results.

This chapter will focus on the recruitment process involving the coordination between third-party providers and an investigative site. In addition, this chapter will explore some retention techniques and tips that can be implemented at the site and/or through third party providers to increase recruitment success and patient retention.

Study Awareness

Study awareness starts from the very beginning of the physician's interest in the study.

The timing of initiation, recruitment, enrollment, study monitoring and final results needs to be communicated to all individuals and entities that will be involved in the study. The lack of timely information sharing can be devastating to a study.

Two crucial pieces that are often overlooked in the beginning of the study are the distribution of the key contact people involved in the study and a timeline that outlines the planned time frame of the study itself. This information is not difficult to obtain, but if not provided can lead to wasteful hours of backtracking through documents, phone messages and emails.

Key contact information should include individuals from the physician through coordinators, marketing personnel, IRB, sponsor, site management organization (SMO) and/or contract research organization (CRO) contacts, etc. Providing phone numbers, addresses and email information eliminates redundancy and provides consistent sources of information. In addition to the contact information, a timeline of events and key dates is a crucial piece of information that should be obtained early in a study program. Timelines should include such items as initiation date, dates advertising and marketing programs will begin, enrollment deadline, site randomization and completion dates. This information can be overlaid against other study timelines, vacation schedules, marketing opportunities and advertising events.

In addition to the site's involvement with managing recruitment activities for a study, the sponsor may elect to hire a third-party provider (i.e., SMO, CRO, patient recruitment vendor, etc.) to facilitate the recruitment process and support the sites. Therefore, it is imperative to the relationship between the third-party provider and the sites to communicate the relationship of the sponsor and the provider as well as the responsibilities of the provider and services to be provided to support the sites. This upfront communication among all parties establishes a positive team relationship and eliminates frustration. Moreover, the third-party provider should outline the project manager's responsibilities, which should include, but not be limited to the following: (1) serve as liaison between sites and sponsor; (2) conduct site feasibility assessments; (3) manage media buys and send media notifications to sites as scheduled.

The use of third-party providers by the sponsor can be advantageous to investigative sites. For example, if there is a common theme the sites are experiencing with the protocol design, the provider can help a sponsor see that an amendment to the protocol may be in order. Individual investigative sites will benefit immensely from the involvement of a third-party provider, because third-party providers, in general, have more bargaining power with the sponsor. It is unwise for a site not to recognize this and use the third-party provider to their advantage.

However, a source of frustration on the site level with the involvement of third-party providers is the unnecessary redundancy of paperwork. For example, a site will complete and submit regulatory documents to the CRO and then be asked to complete the same set of documents again for the SMO. With the use of an established study contact list, the two organizations should be able to communicate clearly and concisely and exchange the information without wasting valuable staff hours at the site level.

Tip

Keep tickler files for all studies in a central file location enabling parties to quickly access important study information.

Marketing/Advertising Focus

Understanding your target audience is a crucial first step in determining the appropriate communication strategy to meet recruitment goals. Defining your target audience's needs and motivations and coupling this information with the study's protocol will aid in the development of an effective message and recruitment strategy. Furthermore, the site must develop metric tracking processes, which will allow for ongoing monitoring of the recruitment strategies and evaluate successes.

Whenever a new study is awarded to a site, the coordinator(s) and/or the marketing department should be notified in respects to whether the site will be implementing their own advertising campaign or whether a company has been hired to produce a national campaign. Oftentimes, the advertising program for a study can be a combination of the above initiatives. However, there can be advantages for a site to be given the opportunity to create and implement its own advertising campaign. The most obvious advantage for the investigative site is the intimate knowledge they have of their local media and community. Every geographic area and town has its own flavor, and this fact is not always reflected in published media ratings (such as Arbitron). If the advertising is going to be completely outsourced, the outsourcing company should contact the site and conduct site feasibility assessments to ascertain venues that have proven success rates. It is important for the outsourcing company to identify the appropriate personnel within the site during their assessment who can speak to the outcome of past recruitment techniques and success rates. Investigative sites that do not have a delegated marketing department tend to benefit from an outsourced advertising campaign. In addition, investigative sites that are in close proximity to one another and/or in urban areas (where media advertising is very expensive) can benefit from a coordinated effort.

Another question that comes up when a sponsor is deciding on its advertising approach is whether to use centralized call center services. The use of centralized call center services has increasingly become more popular over the last several years. An advantage of utilizing a call center is having a person answering calls 24 hours a day, seven days a week. This is something a site cannot accomplish without external support. Another advantage to the sponsor is that a call center can compile analytical data such as cost per call and referral tracking information. A distinct disadvantage to the call center is that they can be impersonal and have limited knowledge of the protocol other than the script they are reading.

If a site is offered the opportunity to conduct a site-specific campaign, there are many steps that should be followed to ensure its success. First and foremost, a site should look to its patient database at the onset of every new study. A patient list should be printed out of patients that fall into the inclusion/exclusion parameters. Ideally, the site should develop a patient letter and submit for IRB approval prior to the onset of enrollment. The letters should be sent out and a follow up phone call made to these patients within the week of their receipt.

Under the HIPAA Privacy Rule, an investigator or a member of his or her staff is allowed to communicate directly with patients without patient authorization and to use the protected health information (PHI) necessary to contact these patients to discuss the option of enrolling in a clinical trial. PHI may also be used to solicit authorizations from a physician's own database. PHI can be used to compose a mailing list of potential study subjects and write to them to request authorization to use their PHI for recruitment. Therefore, the investigator can send a letter to his or her patients asking for written authorization to use their PHI for recruitment purposes; an authorization form should be included in the letter. It is acceptable for an investigator to keep information on potential study subjects for future use, but he or she should obtain a pre-research authorization from each potential subject. The investigator must also be careful not to use the PHI in this database for any purpose not covered in the pre-research authorization. Some investigators now routinely ask their patients to sign these authorization forms when they come in for an office visit.

After database patient letters and phone calls are completed, the site needs to develop radio, newspaper and TV ads. These ads should be eye-catching, protocol-specific and not too wordy.

Tip

When at all possible, it is mutually beneficial to use the doctors' names and even pictures of them within the content of the ad. This is especially important to convey trust to the community. A potential patient in the community or surrounding area generally recognizes the name and/or picture of the doctor. This recognition lends the study credibility. The same holds true for TV ads.

Tip

One innovative method that a site can use to keep costs down for TV production is to have the production company come into the site and film footage of the principal Investigators talking in general terms about certain conditions (i.e., arthritis, osteoporosis, etc.). Additional footage can be taken of the office, staff, DEXA in use, etc. When a study comes up that would benefit from TV advertising, the site can then add voice-over that includes the study specifics. The toll-free phone number should be displayed throughout the duration of the commercial.

External Marketing Strategies

Once a site has identified the target audience and developed a marketing campaign, there are several external marketing strategies that a site can consider for implementation. Some external strategies include, but are not limited to, print, radio and TV advertisements.

Once IRB approval is obtained for the advertisements, then the site can collect media buying information, which will include advertisement availability. With respect to TV advertising, depending on the budget and geographic area, some prime-time spots can be bought within a package. Because all research points to the female in the household as being the major decision maker, it is a good idea to buy spots during morning talk shows such as *Regis and Kelly* and *The Morning Show*. Using the sites' doctor's names and office location again adds credibility and trust.

In addition to using site-specific print and TV ads, another idea is to use the same voice in radio ads. By utilizing this method, the audience again gets the message that this is a credible site and feels comfortable in making the call.

There are many creative and inventive ideas that a site can use to attract its target population. Sometimes trial and error is inevitable. It is essential for a site to be flexible. Change the things that do not work, and do not be afraid to think out of the box and get creative. To put it simply, what works for one site in one geographic location, will not necessarily work for another. The following ideas have proven successful for one rural Pennsylvania site:

Tips

- Display posters in local grocery stores, pharmacies, clinics, motor vehicle bureaus, unemployment offices, health clubs and senior centers.
- Advertise on medicine bags distributed in pharmacy chains (these are the bags that the pharmacies use to distribute the customer's prescription). Ads strategically placed on these bags hit a very large percentage of target patient population(s).
- Full-page color inserts in the local newspaper.
- Full-page color ads in smaller, private papers such as *The Shoppers Guide*, *Fifty-Five Plus*, and *Pennysaver*.
- Distribute coupons in home mailers such as ValuePak.
- Conduct external mailings utilizing a mailing house such as City List.
- Place Internet postings on all relevant sites. For example, a Crohn's study can be listed on the National Crohn's Foundation web site. Other web sites include www.clinicaltrials.org and the sites' own web site.
- Mailings can be done directly from national foundations (i.e., The National Psoriasis Foundation will mail letters directly to the chosen geographic area about the study).
- Ads placed in disease-specific newsletters (i.e., lupus ad for a study can be placed in the National Lupus Foundation Newsletter in region nearest to site).
- Information and brochures can be provided to other physicians in the area informing them about the study. In some cases, it is beneficial to hold an open house with food and beverages and invite other physicians to hear about opportunities for their patients.

- Hold an open house for the public and have a question and answer period on "Everything You Ever Wanted to Know About Clinical Research."

- Use free cable public access channels to advertise new studies.

- Fax news releases to all newspaper contacts and follow up to make sure they are placed in a timely manner.

- Invite a local TV personality to do a segment on enrolling and/or upcoming studies. One idea is to have them shoot footage of several different studies throughout an interview so they can air them at different times. When possible, have the TV station notify the site when they are going to air these segments so enough staff can be on hand to field phone calls.

- Have a physician or other knowledgeable staff member available for local radio talk shows.

- Participate in health fairs. Offer a service such as a heel scan for osteoporosis, or a finger prick for cholesterol at no charge. This will generate interest in your booth and afford you the opportunity to talk about other relevant studies to the potential patient.

- When at all possible, bring a door prize or give-aways to the health fair. Some ideas for door prizes are T-shirts, sweatshirts or hats emblazoned with site information (branding opportunity). Also, many drug representatives have give-away items available such as night-lights, jar and door openers, etc.

- Find out what local chapters of specific indications have meetings in your community (i.e., Leukemia Society of America). Call and ask if a representative from your site can attend the meeting and speak briefly about the study. Hand out brochures.

- Join the local Chamber of Commerce and/or Convention Center. This will enable the site to have its name in a directory listing, will enhance networking and will keep the site abreast of upcoming advertising opportunities.

- Billboards are a very popular medium in some geographic locations. Billboard advertising coupled with a mixture of other media can be very effective.

- Advertise in religious newsletters (i.e., church, temple, etc.).

- Call local hospitals and Veterans' Hospitals/Homes. Ask about getting an opportunity to reach their patient population. Provide incentives to residents/nurses for qualified referrals.

- Call local clinics and ask if there is an opportunity to do a patient information session.

- Contact local universities. Sometimes there is an opportunity to broadcast information on their private network.

- Contact local health clubs and offer to do an informative workshop (i.e., Arthritis and Exercise). This would be mutually beneficial and give the site the opportunity to talk about available studies.

- Become acquainted with the writers for the Health or Lifestyle section of local papers. Ask them to come in and interview the doctors and report on new and exciting research. Request many extra copies and display them in the waiting area.

- Personalize patient database letters when at all possible. Instead of addressing them "Dear Patient" try using the patient's name, "Dear Ms. Smith."

- Keep enrollment lists of prior studies handy to cross reference when enrolling for a similar study.

- Keep a list of the DNQs (Do Not Qualify's). A patient who does not qualify for one study may be a perfect candidate for another.

- Immediately after first contact with potential patients, send them a "thank you for your interest" letter.

- Display a creative bulletin board in the lobby or waiting area of patient success stories (no names please).

- Create an informative voice message while patients are on hold.

Importance of Metric Tracking in Evaluating Marketing Strategies

As displayed in the previous ideas and tips, there are many marketing strategies a site can implement regardless of the amount of advertising dollars allocated in the budget. The most important aspect in evaluating and planning marketing strategies within a site is the ability to track outcome metrics of implemented strategies. Sites should implement an onsite tracking system, which would allow the sites to evaluate which advertising venues were used for which protocol, how much was spent, how many phone calls were generated from each medium and, ultimately, how many patients were enrolled. This level of tracking provides support to the site's recruitment plans submitted to the sponsor and/or third party provider for consideration. Whether the site is enrolling in a low-budget study, or has the support of a national campaign, it is the site's responsibility to utilize as many strategies as possible.

For individual sites that do not have dedicated marketing personnel or the support of a national campaign offered through a third-party provider, there are some shortcuts that can assist them in the advertising process.

Tip

- Use IRB-approved ads from the sponsor or third-party provider with the addition of site-specific information vs. creating your own.
- Have contracts in place with local media and any credit applications/ signatures authorized prior to the beginning of the study.
- Confirm the dollar amount allocated to the site for advertising.
- Conduct a search within the practice's database and allocate a few staff members to call patients personally.

Personalize the Study Experience

Follow-Up and Follow Through

A site has one chance to make a first impression. The goal is to generate patients' interest in the study so that they respond to the mailing either through returning the reply card or calling the site and/or call center, if a call center is used. As the sites begin to receive the reply cards, the sites must be diligent in contacting these potentially interested patients. Ideally, no more than 24 to 48 hours should pass from the time the site receives a patient's reply card or phone call until the time a staff member from the site contacts that patient. If a third party is involved, it is essential to have that direct line of communication already in place to ensure that the referrals are received by the designated person and do not get lost. Moreover, it is important for the site to allow for flexibility in staff scheduling. This flexibility allows for the site to contact interested patients outside daytime hours who are not available to take calls during the day due to their work schedule.

Tip

When possible, sites should arrange for staff to work flexible hours. Staff who work evening hours from 6:00-9:00PM are more successful in reaching patients and scheduling them for an appointment. In addition, patients appreciate the time the site has taken to accommodate them.

Listen to the Story

It has been estimated by Sarah Ebner and Joseph Sameh (Investigator Support Services and Phone Screen) that as many as 20% of prospective study patients do not keep their appointments. Such a large number may be attributed to the de-personalization of the initial call process. A patient that calls into a call center or directly to the site must be handled with dignity and compassion.

Once a site staff member has contacted the patient, he or she needs to be ready and willing to hear that patient's story. The patients do not want to feel as though they are being read to off of a script. The patient is confiding to that staff member a very personal subject—their health or a loved one's health. Fear, desperation and anxiety can often be heard, and it is important to be sympathetic and take the time to hear what the patient is saying. This is the site's chance to convey trust and compassion. If the time is taken to express concern, the patient will feel good about scheduling and keeping the appointment. The site must try to be as flexible as possible when scheduling an appointment. Some patients must absolutely work around their job schedules, or, in some cases, only certain times of day will work for them.

Tip

> Whenever possible, the site must allow patients some independence in choosing their day and time of appointment. Patients will be more likely to keep their appointment because, among other things, they will feel validated.

Know Your Patients

It is important for the entire study team to remember that there are different types of patients who participate in a study with different motivations. Because motivations and populations are different throughout the varied geographic markets, the recruitment, retention and appeal of the study need to be under constant review. Modifications need to be made and adjustments expected.

Tip

> Tailor your questionnaire form to ask why the patient is interested in participating in a clinical research study.

If the site understands the patient's motivations from the beginning, a more fulfilling relationship can be established. Individual sites would do well to remember that if a third-party provider is involved in the study, they have the resources, expertise and research available to them to assist the sites in better understanding their patient's motivations and concerns. Whether the patient is motivated due to desperation, martyrdom, financial compensation or lack of medical assistance available to them, a cooperative working environment and a mutual respect and understanding of each team member's strengths and contributions will ensure successful patient recruitment, retention and well being.

Transportation

One obstacle a patient may have in scheduling an appointment is transportation or their ability to get to the study site. There are a number of methods a site can implement to alleviate this obstacle for patients. One tactic is for a site to set up an account with its local cab company. Negotiate the best price possible and be sure the cab company knows that your patients may need a little extra time getting in and out of their home, office and/or the cab. This method works well for patients who have no other means of transportation and live fairly nearby to the site. For patients who live too far from a local cab company, another option is a local van service that specializes in transporting patients to and from their doctor's offices. A site can check the local yellow pages under "Van Service" and/or "Health Ride." After using this type of service, our site found the offer of transportation to needy patients so much in demand, that we hired an exclusive driver and van. Certainly an endeavor such as this needs to be well thought out, but we found that we were able to include an invaluable number of patients in our studies by offering them this service.

Tip

If offering transportation services is not feasible for a site, then simply offering a gasoline gift card to help pay for gas or brainstorming with a patient about what public transportation may work for them will also be helpful. To this extent, a site should have on hand all local bus, subway, and train schedules to assist the patient.

How Are You Doing?

An alert and compassionate front desk staff can make a big difference in the patient's experience and compliance. On-site opportunities to assist in making the patients' visits as comfortable as possible should be established. Sometimes when patients are enrolled in studies, they have to spend many hours at the site for different reasons. In order for a patient not to feel forgotten about, site personnel can routinely do a room check. If a patient is waiting a long time for the doctor, study coordinator, blood work, etc., have a staff member visit and see how they can facilitate the process. Usually, an offer of a beverage or something to eat is a comforting gesture. It is helpful if a site can keep on hand some extra orange juice, muffins, crackers, etc.

If possible, establishing a domicile room for the comfort of the patient helps to make their visit more pleasant. Keeping on hand several decks of cards, board games and current magazines as well as a selection of television channels can make a patient's visit not only tolerable, but also enjoyable. If there are several patients biding their hours at the same time, they may also like to engage in a game together. Parents, or in some instances grandparents caring for their grandchildren, may benefit from on site daycare.

Tip

A site can celebrate certain visits by giving the patients a thank you token. Our site utilizes T-shirts, hats or sweatshirts emblazoned with the site's logo and name as thank you items. Finally, a very simple, heartfelt "thank you" is always appreciated.

Summary

There are many different ways investigative sites achieve success when participating in clinical research studies. Working with a third-party provider does not mean the investigative site is a passive participant in the research program. Both sides need to assess and acknowledge strengths within this partnership and assign responsibilities accordingly. The investigative site must be an active participant in ensuring that critical aspects of the study are properly communicated and timing of key events are coordinated. Focus in advertising and patient experience, whether working alone or with a third-party provider, ensures that the patient sees and hears a consistent message. The most satisfying result is the patients' feeling they benefited from participating in the research program.

Key Takeaways

- Responsibility and success of patient recruiting rest with both the third-party provider and the investigative site.
- Focused advertising leads to greater efficiencies in screening patients.
- Look for branding opportunities in local area markets.
- Patients overall experience from first contract through study awareness is a key to retention.

References

1. *A Guide to Patient Recruitment: Today's Best Practices and Proven Strategies.* CenterWatch, Inc. Diana Anderson et al. 2001, page 163.

Author Biography

Pam Kivitz-Keenan
Director of Patient Recruitment, Altoona Center for Clinical Research

Pamela Kivitz-Keenan is the Director of Patient Recruitment for the Altoona Center for Clinical Research, a comprehensive rheumatology practice in western Pennsylvania. Ms. Kivitz-Keenan is responsible for all aspects of patient recruitment at the Center and is responsible for the development and implementation of many new and innovative recruitment and retention practices. Altoona Center for Clinical Research, with Dr. Alan J. Kivitz at the helm, has participated in hundreds of clinical research studies and often succeeds as "top enroller."

Ms. Kivitz-Keenan is professionally and personally committed to improving study patient experiences and the general publics' perception of clinical research. Her community involvement includes membership in the Blair County Chamber of Commerce, Blair County Convention Center and Visitor's Bureau, and Founding Member of The Center for Adoption Education of Central Pennsylvania. Ms. Kivitz-Keenan also is a founding partner of Doctor's Orders, LLC.

A graduate of the State University of Albany, Ms. Kivitz-Keenan holds a B.A. in psychology and is a Master of Social Work candidate. Ms. Kivitz-Keenan has extensive experience in the social service field. She worked at Spence-Chapin Services for Families and Children, providing adoption outreach education and counseling services for all members of the adoption triad. She also worked with a pilot program for emotionally challenged children in a group home setting, Sponsored by the Mental Health Association of Nassau County and for the United Synagogue of America as a program coordinator/developer.

A Patient Recruitment Rescue Campaign from Contracting to Completion: A Case Study

Melynda Geurts, MS, D. Anderson & Company
Brian R. Oscherwitz, MBA, CCRC, Biovail Technologies, Ltd.

Objectives

- Identify current and potential recruitment challenges (obstacles), which can hinder enrollment.
- Evaluate initiative(s) outcomes to determine effectiveness and continuation of initiative(s).
- Develop contingency plan based on perceived enrollment challenges at the onset of a recruitment program to minimize potential obstacles and/or barriers.
- Establish mechanisms and rationale for tracking and evaluating program metrics to determine effectiveness and success rate.

Introduction

Medical advancements bring more stringent study designs, thus narrowing the scope of the available patient population. Hence, patient recruitment service providers (PRSPs) will be challenged with redefining their recruitment tactics, including international service offerings, in order to coincide with the changing recruitment landscape. In addition, within the last five years, sponsor companies have taken a more proactive approach regarding the implementation of recruitment programs. Still, a large amount of recruitment programs are rescue. The following case study will focus on a rescue campaign, which consisted of ongoing contingency planning, program outcomes and lessons learned.

Case Study Therapeutic Specifics

The project study involved two phase III research protocols evaluating the efficacy and safety of an opioid-like oral analgesic in patients with osteoarthritis (OA) of the hip and/or knee and OA of the knee. One hundred U.S. research sites were challenged with enrolling a combined 300 patients over a four-month period. (Please note that this recruitment campaign was conducted before the HIPAA Privacy Rule went into effect.)

The sponsor contracted with a contract research organization (CRO) to assist in facilitating enrollment completion. However, the sponsor and CRO encountered several enrollment obstacles that prevented the timelines from being met. These obstacles included a seven-day washout period (must stop current medications), laboratory criteria and a placebo offering, to name a few. Therefore, the sponsor and CRO found themselves behind target.

It was at that time that the sponsor decided to contract with a PRSP to develop, implement and manage a rescue recruitment campaign. The PRSP was challenged with stimulating enrollment to complete a total of 300 randomized patients within four months. In addition, this contract possessed a risk-sharing arrangement, should milestones throughout the contract not have been met by the PRSP.

Challenges

The PRSP was faced with several challenges throughout the contractual period, which hindered the success of some of the employed recruitment initiatives. These challenges included the following:

- Determining which recruitment strategies fit which sites
- Large patient requirement, short period of time to recruit them
- Competing studies
- Program implementation timeline
- Risk associated with the advertising "blitz"
- Lack of site referral follow-up
- Screen failures
- Estimated per-patient cost vs. actual per-patient cost
- Funding limitations

Determining Which Recruitment Strategies Fit Which Sites

There are three common schools of thought in the industry when it comes to extending assistance to sites in their endeavor to recruit patients through the various forms of advertising media.

1. Site personnel know best how to utilize advertising funds locally to maximize patient recruitment potential.

2. Centralized patient recruitment generates the greatest activity in the shortest period of time. It also allows the sponsor to recognize the greatest advertising efficiencies through centralized ad development, approval, planning and placement while taking advantage of the PRSP's expertise and resources.
3. Sites will meet maximum potential through a mix of both local and centralized patient recruitment assistance.

While there is no right or wrong philosophy that one can apply to all sites, the challenge facing the project team in this case was the necessity to marry the right method with the right site while regulating the influx of referrals such that patient overload was minimized. With 100 active sites, it was necessary to carefully evaluate each relative to clinical trial experience, staffing level, available patient base and local media costs along with numerous other variables.

Competing Studies
The PRSP was charged with the responsibility of randomizing 300 patients over a four-month interval for two 1,000-patient trials. At the same time, three other phase III OA trials requiring similar patient populations were in direct competition. As a result of these competing studies, typical recruitment challenges were compounded by reduced availability of experienced investigators and a significant reduction in the eligible patient population. In addition, feasibility data indicated that recruitment leverage was most probably affected due to competing trials offering more competitive investigator budgets.

Program Implementation Timeline
Given a recruitment program of this magnitude, it takes a minimum of four to six weeks to roll out the campaign. Since this program was a four-month rescue program, the benefit that the PRSP provided to the Sponsor is the ability to implement the program in phases. A phased implementation allows for certain initiatives to be launched within two to three weeks of execution. However, once the contract was executed, the sponsor requested that the PRSP place media buys within that same week. There was no time to conduct site feasibilities to determine historically, effective recruitment venues. The selected sites to receive advertising support were provided to the PRSP by the sponsor and CRO. All requested media buys were completed; however, the PRSP did not have the appropriate time needed to evaluate placements.

Risk Associated with the Advertising "Blitz"
The advertising "blitz" is a common strategy utilized to generate a great deal of patient referral activity over a short span of time. However, this strategy is not one that can be sustained for any length of time in the majority of patient recruitment campaigns since it quickly becomes a strain on the advertising budget. Due to the accelerated startup of the campaign and the

consequent inability of the PRSP to fully evaluate placements, the employment of the advertising blitz executed near the beginning of this recruitment program did not have the full impact anticipated. This subsequently proved to be a detrimental factor limiting to some extent, future options available for the remainder of the campaign.

Lack of Site Referral Follow-Up

At the time the PRSP became involved in the study, it was observed by the PRSP that some of the sites were losing momentum. This lack of momentum contributed to the lack of referral follow-up experienced by the PRSP from the sites. Until certain stopgap measures were put in place by the PRSP and the sponsor/CRO, the lack of referral follow-up from the sites affected the achievement of the PRSP's contractual goal.

Recruitment Obstacles: Screen Failures and Estimated Per-Patient Cost vs. Actual Per-Patient Cost

Based upon certain study criteria and the side effects experienced by some participants, the average screen fail ratio for the studies was 38.8%. This was 5% higher than predicted. The recruitment funnel was estimated from the predicted screen fail ratio. With the actual screen fail ratio running higher than predicted, this was an unforeseen challenge, which affected the rate of enrollment at large, not to mention the outcomes of the recruitment initiatives.

In addition, the actual per-patient cost also affected the rate of enrollment. Historically for an osteoarthritis trial, the average cost per randomized patient ranges from $1,000-$1,500 per patient. The recruitment budget was based on these historical cost averages. However, when you factor in the actual screen fail ratio, the actual cost per randomized patient was $2,100 per patient, which affected the overall recruitment budget and statistical outcomes from recruitment initiatives.

Funding Limitations

With a firmly established budget, the sponsor, PRSP and CRO were forced to utilize funds in the most disciplined, innovative and efficient ways possible. For this reason it was necessary to closely monitor metrics, develop means of maximizing responsiveness to data received, and to take advantage of patient recruitment opportunities that often pass by sponsors unnoticed, such as referrals not contacted and referrals lost to follow-up.

Program Elements

The recruitment plan included a comprehensive, multi-faceted program, which required adherence to very stringent timelines. The plan included the following strategies, which will be described in detail:

- Site feasibility
- Site support recruitment materials
- Direct mail
- Media planning/buying
- Call center support services
- Site conference calls
- Monthly newsletters

Site Feasibility

The key to a successful recruitment campaign hinges on the relationship one develops with research center personnel, especially the study coordinator. This relationship starts during the initial call between the PRSP and the research center staff, typically the study coordinator or patient recruitment manager, during the site feasibility call. It is through the calls that the PRSP is able to ascertain the exact needs of each individual site and tailor the recruitment program to meet the site's needs. Overall, this feasibility questionnaire assists the PRSP in establishing recruitment benchmarks, which allows for proactive evaluation of the site's performance.

Site Support Recruitment Materials

As indicative with the majority of recruitment campaigns, there needs to be a balance between internal and external recruitment strategies. Research sites are selected based on their historical enrollment metrics as well as what they predict for the study at hand. Therefore, as a PRSP, it is imperative not to underestimate the importance of providing site support recruitment materials to facilitate enrollment within the site's patient population, not to mention their communities. A site support recruitment packet can include a variation or all of the following tools: poster, fliers, brochure, physician-to-patient letter, physician-to-physician letter and inclusion/exclusion study criteria pocket cards. A description of how each of these pieces was employed among the sites is stated below.

The display poster was displayed in the waiting room and/or the exam room of the research facilities as well as the fliers. Moreover, some sites mailed a copy of the flier with the billing statements to their patients. Sites mailed the physician-to-patient letter to their internal database of potential participants to generate study interest. The PRSP identified area rheumatologists and other family practitioners that potentially had access to the osteoarthritis patient population to generate possible patient referrals through the mailing of the physician-to-physician letter. The study specific brochures were also displayed in the waiting room and/or used in a patient mailing as well. The "quick reference" criteria pocket cards, which list the inclusion and exclusion criteria of the study on one side and the visit flow chart on the reverse side, were made available to the investigators and/or study coordinators to identify potential candidates as they presented for an appointment.

Direct Mail

The PRSP implemented and distributed a 38,000-piece, targeted direct mail campaign. Recipients of the direct mail were identified through the PRSP's internal database as well as through geographically matched (to the sites) individuals through external clearinghouses. Individuals obtained through clearinghouses have self-reported their disease or ailment or self-reported on behalf of a family member. Conducting a targeted (criteria specific) direct mail campaign typically yields a 3%–4% call response rate.

To obtain this response rate, the direct mail piece was designed as a tri-fold piece with a reply card allowing the individual to fill out their personal information and to receive a study brochure. Designing the direct mail in this way gives the interested individual two calls of action: (1) complete the reply card to receive the study brochure; or (2) call the centralized call center to pre-screen for the study. This direct mail campaign was supported through a centralized call center, which will be described in detail in the coming sections.

Media Planning/Buying

Based on the feedback received during the site feasibility assessments, the PRSP's ongoing contact with the sites and the PRSP's historical metrics, the PRSP developed a detailed media plan to support the markets represented through the research site's location. The media planning and buying for this case study were centrally managed, but were locally placed within the site's geographic market, with print and radio advertising being utilized.

The sites were given the option to field their own calls from advertisements placed, or the calls from the advertisements could be routed through the call center. Throughout the study, the PRSP evaluated each advertisement placement to ascertain the level of effectiveness prior to additional advertisements being placed.

Call Center Support Services

All recruitment strategies in this case study were supported through a centralized call center. The call center was operational throughout the study, and individuals were able to access the system 24 hours a day, 7 days a week. The success with utilizing a call center is in the design of the screening questionnaire and communicating the rationale to the sites as to why certain criteria questions were or were not asked.

The sponsor and PRSP developed the questionnaire in conjunction with one another. This process allowed the sponsor to identify specific criteria questions that should not be overlooked as well as identify criteria questions, which need to be determined by the investigator.

All responses from the implemented recruitment strategies, which were supported by the call center, were pre-screened for study participation. If the individual pre-screen qualified, then their completed questionnaire was faxed to the appropriate research site for follow-up within 48 hours of notification. Once the research sites received the referral, then the PRSP followed up on each referral to obtain referral outcomes. This information was then reported back to the sponsor on a weekly basis.

Site Conference Calls

In a rescue campaign, the PRSP's opportunity to engage with multiple sites at the same time is through site conference calls. These calls were implemented during this program to create buy-in into the recruitment program and to generate an open forum for discussions regarding successes, obstacles and other recruitment challenges the sites were experiencing throughout the course of the study. The investigator, study coordinator, sponsor and CRO were invited to participate in these calls. There were two calls conducted over the four-month contract.

The "kick-off" call allows the PRSP to introduce themselves to the sites, describe the relationship between the Sponsor, CRO and PRSP, and to describe the components of the recruitment program. The PRSP takes time to explain how the program will roll out and how the sites can obtain the maximum benefit from participating in the program.

The second call was conducted at 2 months into the program. This call served as an open forum roundtable for sites to share their recruitment successes and/or challenges. Typically, the PRSP will invite a site that has implemented various recruitment tactics with success to present their techniques to others on the call. Moreover, these calls are a viable opportunity for the sponsor and/or CRO to learn of potential and actual recruitment obstacles, whether it is related to protocol design and/or research personnel, etc.

Monthly Newsletters

The PRSP developed and distributed study-related newsletters to the sites monthly. These newsletters served as an excellent communication tool to the sites as it kept the sites abreast of the study progress and outcomes. Stories and briefs included top study enrollers, interviews with sites that had a positive outcome from recruitment initiative(s), recruitment tips, protocol updates and CRO/sponsor updates. Study newsletters also provide benefit to the study through facilitating awareness about the study among the research staff. Moreover, it establishes a team approach among all parties, as it keeps the sites informed regarding study progress.

Outcomes

The previously described recruitment program was designed to generate 300 randomized patients within a four-month rescue period. Overall, the program generated a total of 4,407 call responses. The breakdown of these responses is depicted in Table 1.[3]

Table 1: Call Response Outcomes

Category	Outcome	Percent of Total Outcome
Total Calls	4,407	
Total Referred	871	20%
Total Scheduled	744	17%
Total Screened	441	10%
No Site in Area	148	3%
Total Disqualified	3,030	69%
Screen Failures	171	4%
Lost to Follow-Up	157	4%
No Shows	30	Less than 1%
Total Randomized	231	5%

Of the 4,407 responses, the results per initiative are outlined in Table 2.[4]

Table 2: Call Response Outcomes

Initiatives	Calls	Referrals	Referral Rate
Print	1,345	501	37%
Direct Mail	550	174	32%
Radio	524	153	29%
TV—3 markets	106	32	30%
Email Notification	16	5	31%

As indicated in Table 2, the two most successful initiatives were print and direct mail, with 1,345 and 550 calls and 501 and 174 referrals, respectively. However, halfway into the contract, the PRSP realized the goal of 300 randomized patients was not going to be achieved. Several factors hindered the predicted success of this campaign. Those factors included certain inclusion/exclusion laboratory criteria, a two-week program implementation, and the lack of referral follow-up, which attributed to the PRSP's lack of success in tracking all PRSP-generated referrals back to the PRSP.

Once realized the goal was not going to be obtained given some uncontrollable factors, the PRSP restructured the recruitment program to include a change in external outreach efforts as well as internal tracking processes.

Given the remaining recruitment budget, the PRSP implemented a different, cost-effective recruitment strategy as well as expanded their print media buys, since print proved to have the highest referral rate. The new strategy identified was utilizing a patient database provider who could identify potential participants given study criteria and site locations. These identified individuals were sent an email notification about the study and were prompted to contact the call center if they were interested in participating in the clinical research study. This initiative proved to be an effective venue for reaching out to individuals who had already at one point opted-in to receive additional information about their disease. This email notification allowed the PRSP to reach out to a highly interested and motivated target population.

The other necessary change within the existing recruitment program was the referral tracking process. At one point within the study, the PRSP was challenged with resolving 140 aging patients. These were patients that had been referred to the site through implemented recruitment strategies, but had not been scheduled for an appointment within two weeks of notification. To address this issue, which had an ultimate impact on the PRSP's contractual goal, the PRSP implemented several tactics. These tactics included referral notification and follow up from the call center, a letter from the Sponsor addressing the urgency and importance of referral follow up and scheduling, and a combined effort between the PRSP and the CRAs to obtain referral resolution from the sites. In addition, the sites were given the option of allowing the call center to schedule these patients once prescreened to try and minimize outstanding contacts and those lost-to-follow-up. With these tactics in place, only 4% of the total responses resulted in lost-to-follow-up. All other referrals were resolved.

Finally, it was at this time, the PRSP and the sponsor agreed that the PRSP would concede their risk share to the Sponsor. Furthermore, based on the cost per randomized patient, the PRSP and the sponsor agreed on a revised enrollment contractual goal of 200 randomized patients. As shown in Table 1, with this revised plan, the PRSP was able to garner 231 randomized patients within the remaining timeline.

Lessons Learned

For every new challenge there is a solution, and with every challenge overcome, there is a lesson learned. From the successful collaboration between the PSRP and sponsor came a series of lessons that can be applied to future patient recruitment endeavors whether they are conceived as a proactive measure or whether they are implemented in the rescue environment.

- Tailor advertising strategy to conform to site needs and capacity
- Ensure advertising expenditures make financial and strategic sense
- Never underestimate the impact of a well-developed call center script

- Arrange for a dedicated project coordinator/project manager
- Don't let referrals languish
- True risk sharing is reciprocal
- Cost containment through metrics

Tailor Advertising Strategy to Conform to Site Needs and Capacity

Prior to ad placement during the course of the project, sites were asked at several junctures what their preferences were with respect to the mode of patient recruitment assistance they wished to receive. The choices were "Centralized Patient Recruitment" through the PRSP or direct funding for "Local Patient Recruitment" whereby the site was entrusted with funds to plan and place its own advertisements within close proximity.

There was also a third option offered; this project utilized an integrated model involving site personnel responding to the PRSP with their placement preferences. This allowed them a choice of the following:

1. Locally placing advertisements independently;
2. Having the PRSP place the ads locally (resulting in cost efficiencies when media placements were "bundled" for the study); or
3. Having the PRSP define the media type, identify the outlet and place the ad for the site.

This model worked very well since it empowered sites experienced enough to know where their patients were, yet allowed for the utilization of the value and expertise provided by the PRSP. This approach also offered a certain amount of comfort to the sponsor who was concerned about the potential for sites unreceptive to PRSP assistance to become displeased if forced to utilize such services. Finally, and by no means of least importance, the integrated model allowed the site to regulate the inflow of prospective patients based on their capacity to adequately process them. This is of key importance for a lean, yet efficient patient recruitment program.

Ensure Advertising Expenditures Make Financial and Strategic Sense

The advertising "blitz" should be employed carefully with the available advertising budget in mind. Considering a hypothetical project, as the available advertising budget becomes smaller and campaign duration becomes longer, the risk factor associated with the "blitz" becomes proportionally higher. The use of this strategy must be carefully considered for projects characterized by both limited advertising budget and extended duration to avoid expending too large a proportion of advertising funds too early in the project. While risky, it is understandable that an advertising "blitz" strategy was employed for this rescue program, as risk is often more acceptable under such conditions. Had a better opportunity to evaluate media placement been possible prior to its implementation the "blitz" could have had its desired effect, and the project may well have met its originally proposed objective.

Never Underestimate the Impact of a Well-Developed Call Center Script

Due to the difficult prospect of recruiting patients while operating in an environment characterized by several competing protocols, it was determined that it would be beneficial to perform an interim reevaluation of the call script utilized to screen patients calling into the call center for eligibility. Organized metric data allowed the project team to collectively identify several of the primary reasons why callers were being disqualified before being directed to the site level for further evaluation. Identified barriers were reevaluated within the context of the basis for the protocol requirements, the protocol objectives, and whether or not there was flexibility in regard to future disqualifications. Identified improvements were then made to the call script, and it was put back into service. This process allowed for the more focused screening of patients suitable for the sponsor's specific protocols. The end result was a screen failure rate (38.8%) closely approximating that of the study overall (39.5%). This signifies the existence of an efficient recruitment system that is not inundating sites with ineligible referrals, but rather is providing them with a tangible source of prospective participants.

Arrange for a Dedicated Project Coordinator/Project Manager

One of the sponsor requirements for this recruitment program was the inclusion of a dedicated project manager (PM). The PM proved to be key to gaining an understanding of the ever-changing dynamics of the project. The role of the PM included daily communication of metrics concerning call center activity, patient scheduling, site screening and patient randomization. In addition, this individual analyzed other metrics pertaining to reasons for disqualification, monitored media buys and worked with sites to develop advertising strategies in coordination with the PRSP and CRO. Without this pivotal resource, the project team would have been blind to the trends necessary to quickly make informed decisions regarding future steps.

Don't Let Referrals Languish

In the process of monitoring patient recruitment metrics, a significant number of referrals were seen to be outstanding; that is, their disposition was yet to be determined. Upon closer investigation, it was determined that the referrals, each representing a potential eligible patient, had not yet been contacted by site personnel for the purpose of scheduling a visit. In any patient recruitment campaign there will be some amount of overload occurring at a subset of sites. Having the appropriate personnel available to perform follow up on outstanding referrals provides an extra measure of recruitment potential, which would otherwise be lost (see Arrange for a Dedicated Project

Coordinator/Project Manager). In addition, the PRSP should be capable of preparing an *aging report*. The function of the aging report is to present the numbers of referrals who have not yet been contacted and for what period of time they have been waiting. Clearly, the longer the referral has to wait to be contacted the less likely he or she is to reach the enrollment stage.

True Risk-Sharing Is Reciprocal

During the course of the rescue campaign, several assumptions on which the project agreement was based were found to be inaccurate. However, all parties involved were experienced professionals and were, therefore, not particularly surprised. There should be an understanding among contracting parties that assumptions are nothing more than educated guesses. Assumptions are almost without exception, replaced with an alternate observed reality as time progresses. Consequently, one of the various skills vital to the development and maintenance of a successful partnership is the ability to offer solutions when confronted with challenges. Since time cannot be reversed and actions cannot be undone, a solution-orientation is what directs us to the best possible outcome in any situation. The PRSP conducting the rescue campaign worked with the sponsor in good faith to maximize patient recruitment outcomes through reduction of the organization's own profit margin while the sponsor agreed to forego an agreed-upon risk sharing credit for the benefit of the program. This reciprocal give-and-take attitude resulted in good will between organizations and increased productivity with regard to patient recruitment objectives.

Cost Containment Through Metrics

Due to sponsor funding limitations, the tracking of metrics became even more critical than it ordinarily would have been in a non-rescue situation. The PRSP-provided metrics, once in place, made it possible to cost effectively develop ad placement strategy and to better understand where referral follow-up was required. Availability of such information could potentially have increased the effectiveness of the advertising "blitz" had it been available at the time the tactic was employed.

Equally important was the idea that the PRSP-provided metrics allowed for the close monitoring of activity on a daily basis, providing the organizational transparency that fosters a high degree of trust between contracting parties. Existence of appropriate metrics not only allows for a heightened awareness of rescue program activity, but also allows for the tracking and verification of PRSP progress and success.

Establishing Metrics

The world we live in today is dominated by a reliance on data. Transmitted in every conceivable way, from every direction to all corners of the world, data constantly stream around us to the extent that one could say we literally live and breathe data. With the rapid proliferation of technology used to provide us with the data we need to make our decisions comes the potential to be lulled into a false sense of security that comes with having access to an almost unlimited supply of information. While in many ways data are meant to help us better understand the world around us, it is important to realize that data can be just as harmful as they can be helpful if managed improperly. For this reason, one must thoughtfully consider the form data will take and the ways in which it will be used. This is particularly true for the organization engaged in a patient recruitment rescue campaign.

In any patient recruitment campaign, data should be thoughtfully organized in the form of *project metrics*. The *metric* is the bridge spanning the gap between raw, unusable information and a basic understanding of the behavior of a particular chosen study parameter. The discriminating sponsor who wishes to keep abreast of recruitment campaign progress will select a PRSP that has a well-developed system for tracking project metrics. Surprisingly, all providers do not have this capability, or they do and it has not been effectively developed. A well-defined process for the collection and reporting of sound project metrics will involve the following components:

- Direct sponsor input and support for the PRSP
- Sponsor support for PRSP at site level
- Positive relationship with sites derived, in part, from the two points above
- User-friendly data collection forms/patient logs
- A standardized metrics template designed with sponsor needs in mind
- Site awareness of an established schedule for data collection and retrieval
- PRSP staff member dedicated to site follow-up, compilation and reporting of patient recruitment data retrieved from sites

The Value of Metrics

While the most basic purpose of project metrics is to monitor the progress of the recruitment campaign, project metrics have a variety of other uses as shown in Table 3.

Project Navigation
The most obvious reason that comes to mind for troubling oneself with the tracking of metrics is *project navigation*. Without a timely, comprehensive characterization of the factors influencing patient recruitment and, therefore, enrollment, the study manager cannot effectively make the informed decisions necessary to "steer" the patient recruitment campaign in the required direction. This does not imply that timely, comprehensive infor-

mation *guarantees* the study manager will evaluate it correctly and choose the appropriate action. However, it certainly does maximize the possibility of doing so.

Table 3: Value in Project Metrics

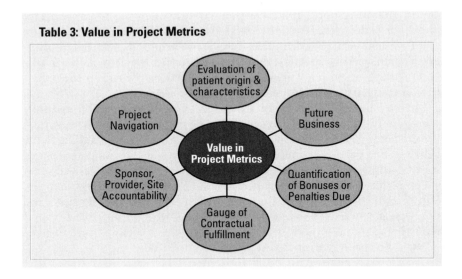

Evaluation of Patient Origin and Characteristics

In order to understand whether or not a patient recruitment campaign is working, one must enact a process for determining whether patients contacting sites or the call center are doing so as a direct result of the patient recruitment campaign strategy or as a result of some other strategy being employed by the sponsor, CRO, or other entity. Under conditions where competing studies sponsored by separate pharmaceutical companies, seeking similar patients are ongoing in parallel, the potential even exists for Company A to pay for a recruitment campaign which funnels patients into the study of competing Company B. Knowing where your potential patients are coming from enables decision makers to make appropriate adjustments to the campaign strategy whether this means modifying the media type, media placement, call center script or entrance criteria, there are a multitude of "fine tuning" controls available to the adept PRSP.

Future Business

In today's complex world, we are asked to place a great deal of faith in technology, disregarding the details and inner workings of the systems we so depend on. For this reason, Sponsors who wish to delve into the workings of the patient recruitment program will be pleased to align themselves with the organization(s) that can provide concrete, credible metrics indicating the level of success achieved during the course of the patient recruitment campaign. This is helpful to the sponsor in gaining a comfort level with regard to control of his or her destiny with respect to study success, and will provide the same individuals with proof of success to rationalize continued use of the centralized patient recruitment concept in the future.

Sponsor, Provider, Site Accountability

Paying close attention to metrics provides stability within the clinical research triumvirate comprising the sponsor (or sponsor designee, i.e., CRO), PRSP and investigative site. Data made available as a result of clearly defined metrics enable prompt identification of patient access-related issues by the PRSP, give the sponsor information on which to base decisions, and when shared with sites, provide them with an indication of how well they are doing in relation to other sites. Reports including such information are often incorporated into project newsletters due to the fact that the information represents ownership of the outcome thereby imparting a sense of pride and/or competition in site personnel boosting performance. Project metrics highlight the result of the work effort expended on the patient recruitment campaign and can provide a direct link to the source of that effort.

Gauge of Contractual Fulfillment

When all is done the question which is inevitably asked is, "How successful was the patient recruitment campaign?" In some instances the answer to this question is not clear, particularly where metrics are unavailable or inconclusive. It is up to the sponsor, in cooperation with the PRSP to develop metrics that correspond to project objectives and contractual obligations in order to fairly determine whether or not these objectives have ultimately been met. While not a matter of trust or distrust, this is simply a matter of good business practice.

Quantification of Bonuses or Penalties Due

In cases where bonuses and penalties are part of the risk-sharing agreement between the sponsor and PRSP, metrics are an absolute requirement in order to fairly honor the terms inherent in such agreements. Whether bonuses and penalties are based on time, call center activity, referrals, patient evaluations, screenings or patients enrolled, fair compensation for rewards earned cannot be made without the benefit of proper supporting metrics.

Summary

As the number of investigational new drug applications and new drug approvals continues to grow, protocol designs become more stringent, and patient availability decreases, the sponsor and PRSP will be faced with a multitude of different recruitment variables from study to study. However, as depicted in this featured case study, there are significant lessons learned, which can be interposed into any recruitment program.

Based on the lessons learned as described in this case study, it is imperative for both the sponsor and PRSP not to lose sight of the impact of the recruitment program from the development of the media plan through the last referral generated. To this end, project metrics were established for the purpose of guiding the campaign while monitoring progress toward overall objectives. Key elements identified, which increased the likelihood of achieving success included never underestimating the impact of a well-developed screening questionnaire and arranging for a dedicated project manager and/or project coordinator with the PRSP.

Finally, the relationship that the Sponsor and PRSP fostered between one another attributed to the team approach given to this study. Although the initial enrollment goal had to be modified, the team approach between the two parties led to positive outcomes for the study overall.

Key Takeaways

- Successful recruitment campaigns hinge on the development and maintenance of positive relations with research center personnel, especially the study coordinator.
- It is important to properly gauge the needs of each site individually, balancing the employment of internal (within a site's patient population) and external recruitment materials, as well as centralized and local recruitment strategies.
- Giving sites multiple options with which they can approach media placement increases the potential for site productivity. Through this integrated approach, the PRSP and site can cooperatively regulate influx of patient referrals to best match site capacity.
- Optimization of media planning and buying is facilitated through the utilization of site feasibility assessments, ongoing contact with sites and PRSP historical metrics.
- The greatest productivity from call center resources can be achieved through the careful development of the call center script.
- Time invested in tracking and follow up for referrals is time well spent.
- PRSP-prepared aging reports are useful in identifying and addressing substantial numbers of unscheduled referrals.
- In the absence of historical information or metric-based guidance, there can be significant risk in deployment of the advertising blitz strategy; this risk is compounded if a recruitment campaign relies on limited funding and/or extended duration.
- Identifying the origin of patients through appropriate metrics enables the PRSP and sponsor to "fine tune" the various strategic "controls" available to the PRSP.

- Project metrics highlight the result of the work effort expended on the patient recruitment campaign and can provide a direct link to the source of that effort.

References

Active Clinical Studies (Active INDs), PhRMA and FDA, 2003.
Enrollment Delays, Surveys of Investigative Sites, CenterWatch, April 2003.
Patient Recruitment Program—Call Response Outcomes, D. Anderson & Company, January—April 2003.
Patient Recruitment Program—Initiative Outcomes, D. Anderson & Company, January—April 2003.

Author Biographies

Melynda Geurts, MS
Senior Vice President of Operations, D. Anderson & Company
Melynda Geurts, MS, is the Senior Vice President of Operations for D. Anderson & Company (DAC), an international, multi-specialty recruitment provider. Ms. Geurts oversees business development, operations and project management for DAC. Additionally, Ms. Geurts coordinates the company's image building and branding efforts throughout the pharmaceutical industry. Moreover, she was a major contributor to *A Guide to Patient Recruitment: Today's Best Practices and Proven Strategies* authored by Diana L. Anderson, Ph.D., and published by CenterWatch in 2001.

Ms. Geurts' expertise in healthcare marketing, coupled with her extensive experience in the field of patient recruitment, provides her with numerous opportunities to present at industry-related conferences and seminars. Her expansive background and experience contribute significantly to the overall success rate of meeting and exceeding patient recruitment goals at D. Anderson & Company.

Brian Oscherwitz
Manager of Clinical Operations and Outsourcing for Research & Development, Biovail Technologies, Ltd.
Brian Oscherwitz is the Manager of Clinical Operations and Outsourcing for Research & Development at Biovail Technologies, Ltd., a Toronto-based pharmaceutical manufacturing company. Mr. Oscherwitz is responsible for operational, contractual, financial and outsourcing oversight for ongoing and planned programs in developmental phases II to IV. This function also encompasses the development of new and long-lasting relationships with external providers such as CROs, central laboratories,

patient recruitment service providers and other specialized clinical research related providers.

Mr. Oscherwitz previously managed the Investigator Services Department at PPD Development, an established CRO leader with an international presence. Responsibilities of this role included development and maintenance of positive Investigator site relations as well as strategic and logistical support for project management activities in all therapeutic areas of involvement. He holds a Master of Business Administration degree, with a concentration in the Management of Technical and Professional Personnel; and a BA in Microbiology from the University of Texas. He is a member of the Association of Clinical Research Professionals (ACRP) and the Drug Information Association (DIA).

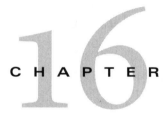

A Progressive Approach to Patient Recruitment and Retention

Kathleen B. Drennan, Chief, Global Marketing and Strategic Business Development, Iris Global Clinical Trial Solutions
Jonathan Bailey, Director of Analytics and Statistics, Iris Global Clinical Trial Solutions

Objectives

- Distinguish the advantages and disadvantages of centralized vs. local (site-based) recruiting
- Identify the challenges facing study sponsors in today's environment
- Understand the importance and value of tracking patients' progress electronically
- Learn how to monitor site performance
- Set benchmarks and project results

Introduction

Patient recruitment and retention for clinical trials are becoming extremely fragmented processes which often leads to missed deadlines for sponsors and studies going into rescue mode. Traditionally, study sponsors have relied on the clinical sites alone to manage this process. The increased regulatory requirements on sites in combination with a shortage of qualified volunteers place a heavy burden on sites leaving little time for the demands of identifying, screening and enrolling qualified volunteers. In addition, the majority of investigative sites are not experienced or resourced to develop and implement the complex community outreach and media programs necessary to find adequate numbers of qualified study patients. More often than not, diligent patient tracking does not occur until the patient is seen at the site for the first screen visit. The majority of pre-qualified patients are lost before the first site visit. Unless a sponsor has mechanisms in place to track the pre-screened or referred patients, it is becoming more and more likely that the study will have insufficient numbers of patients entering the randomization queue.

The diagram below depicts the evolution in the strategies for recruitment and retention, beginning with the more speculative approach on the left. For multi-center studies this represents a somewhat random approach in that each site is left to its own level of competency to develop local strategy and tactics specific to recruiting and retaining patients. Indeed, the entire study can be held hostage by the least productive sites and spiral into study extensions and increased costs. For larger, difficult-to-recruit studies, this site-based approach rarely works as planned. With no central management system in place to track referrals and manage the program, the ability to leverage information for the next phase of the trial and demonstrate return on investment is unlikely.

The second level is more evolved, and a number of study sponsors are having success committing to a more "centralized" approach to addressing the recruitment deficiencies using site-alone based programs. This level represents a central management focus incorporating central patient screening and referral, utilizing shared media defined by targeted messaging, and casting a wide net over the defined patient population. The economies of scale gained by an evolved and less speculative approach can outweigh the upfront costs for such a program.

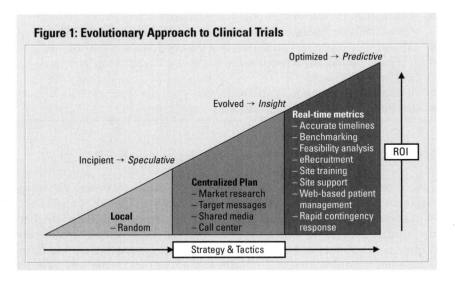

Figure 1: Evolutionary Approach to Clinical Trials

The real promise lies in the optimized and more predictive approach to management of the entire recruitment and retention program within a given clinical trial. In order to reach this level it is imperative to develop a comprehensive program measuring critical activities, benchmarks and patient movement through the trial, in real time. We believe that if "you cannot measure, you cannot manage" any program, and this surely holds true for the complexities of successfully completing a complex clinical trial. In addition, this evolved approach allows the important data captured in the recruitment process to be leveraged in the next phase of trials, which could reduce the time and costs of future trials.

The case studies in this chapter will address common issues related to centralized vs. site-based recruitment and retention. Centralized recruitment has different connotations, including simply an advertising-centric approach. For the purposes of this chapter the term centralized recruitment is defined as an "end-to-end" approach inclusive of strategic planning, market research and creative development, shared media, central data capture and analysis, site modeling and support, and call center screening and referral.

Centralized vs. Site-Based Recruiting

How can study sponsors be certain they will be able to recruit and retain the required number of patients within the desired time frame? This is one of the most common and critical decisions that sponsors face in the planning stages of a clinical trial. Sponsors must decide:

- Do the sites have access to enough patients who will qualify for the study?
- If not, are they capable of gaining enough patients through local advertising on their own in the time frame allotted?
- Do they have the staff and expertise to manage an advertising campaign and track the results?
- Are they able to effectively track each prospective study candidate and follow up with reminder calls, study education materials and additional tools needed to retain patients throughout the process?

If the study team has recent experience recruiting patients for the same condition with similar protocol inclusion/exclusion criteria, they can use that information to project how many volunteers will be needed to fill the trial. Without recent experience, the sponsor is often recruiting blind—at least until the trial has progressed for several months.

Experience has shown that sites tend to be overly optimistic when estimating the number of patients they can enroll. This miscalculation can significantly extend the time required for recruitment which translates directly into lost revenue.

Site-based recruiting is done at the local level with each site recruiting from their patient database or physician practice. Often the sponsor will offer each site an advertising budget to place local ads in order to find additional patients. There are sites dedicated to clinical trial conduct that have experience with their local population and know which newspapers or radio stations to use for advertising information about a clinical trial. However, the majority of clinical sites do not have that capability or experience.

Centralized recruiting works by using a central recruitment and retention management team to

1. Plan and develop strategy
2. Implement community outreach and national advertising programs
3. Manage the process
4. Track the referred volunteers and enrolled patients

The team also includes a dedicated patient interaction center to take calls from volunteers across the country, pre-screen them and refer them to the closest site to their address. More advanced call centers will also set appointment times and send out welcome packages to the volunteers to engage them quickly and educate them about the clinical trial. The advertising used for recruitment includes a 1-800 number to the call center that can be used nationwide. When the sites advertise on their own, each must develop advertising with their local number printed on it. This makes site-based radio and television much more expensive, since different spots and creative pieces have to be made for each site.

More advanced centralized recruiting companies use a data collection and tracking system to bring together media information, patient demographic information, site visit information, patient status and other metrics to track the progress of the recruitment effort. This enables the study team to monitor patient progress from the initial phone contact to the final visit (or disqualification). These metrics are also used to quickly evaluate media performance and make regular adjustments to the media mix for each market. This significant advantage of centralized recruitment allows the sponsor to know precisely what is going on across all sites and make appropriate adjustments as needed.

The decision to adopt site-based recruiting vs. centralized recruiting depends on a number of factors. Each of these needs to be carefully weighed in order make an informed decision:

- How many randomized patients are required?
  - Studies sponsored by pharmaceutical and biotech companies requiring a large number of study volunteers (>300 randomized patients) have an advantage if supported by a centralized team that includes a call center, creative expertise, patient tracking system and study management staff. If the study population is hard to reach or the protocol is difficult, a centralized recruitment approach can be used for studies requiring as few as 75 randomized patients.
- How many sites are selected for the study?
  - Larger studies with more than 10 sites are more conducive to the centralized approach. Significant economies of scale are gained by using a uniform set of creative advertising for all

sites, a central call center to pre-screen and refer all volunteers, and a central management of the process across all sites. Other advantages will be made clear later in the chapter.

- How difficult is the population to reach?
    - If the eligible population is relatively small and difficult to find, a centralized campaign using mass media may be cost-prohibitive. In these instances, there may be opportunities for national outreach through local health agencies or national disease organizations. A "trimmed down" centralized approach may be warranted if the study requires a large sample of patients or if the study protocol is challenging (high drop-out rate). In these cases, it is imperative that the study team keep the patients engaged and active given the difficulty and expense of finding them. This can be achieved more easily with central call center support (reminder calls, postcards, educational materials, etc...).
- How healthy and independent is the study population?
    - Some clinical trials are designed for patients with more extensive disease or severe medical conditions. These patients often must be recommended for enrollment by their physician or surgeon. In these cases, it is the physician who has to be made aware of the new treatment and offered educational materials and information about the trial. Mass advertising (television, radio, etc...) is rarely used under these circumstances. Generally placement of trial information in medical journals, clinical trial listing services, is a common vehicle for getting the word out.
- How stringent is the inclusion/exclusion criteria?
    - If the inclusion/exclusion criteria are going to exclude over half of the disease population, a centralized advertising campaign with a very specific message can be effective. For example, if the population is people with type 2 diabetes, but the protocol requires that they be untreated and recently diagnosed, the advertising/outreach message can effectively reach eligible volunteers if these criteria are included in the advertisements, flyers, etc.
- What are the revenue estimates for the new drug, provided it is approved by the FDA?
    - This issue is often overlooked by clinical teams who are more apt to be focused on the research itself and less cognizant of the market value of the drug once it is approved. If the market potential is high and there are other competitors in the same space, time-to-market is a significant consideration. Some estimate of the market potential should be made to determine how important it is to reach approval quickly. Centralized recruitment will almost always accelerate the recruitment process.

- How competitive is the marketplace for the drug?
  - Pharmaceutical companies are often competing for the same patients, and the race for approval of a new medication can be fast and furious. If the competition is fierce and the drug has a high potential market value upon approval, a centralized approach using extensive advertising and outreach is generally warranted. Sponsors should not allow slow recruitment to drag down the approval process in this case.
- What are the cost differences (centralized vs. site-based)?
  - Ultimately, the decision usually comes down to cost vs. value. The study sponsor must weigh the costs of site-based recruitment vs. centralized and take into consideration the pros and cons of each approach, keeping in mind that time delays usually end up being more costly than costs of a centrally managed program.

Other considerations include the countries in which the study is being conducted, the recruiting proficiency and experience level of the clinical sites, and the sociological make-up of the study population. AIDS and Alzheimer's patients can be particularly difficult to monitor; they require special attention to keep them engaged in the specifics of the study protocol. Every study is different, and each will offer a unique assortment of recruitment and retention challenges.

Funnel Estimates

To effectively decide on the best approach, an astute clinical team will develop a "funnel" to estimate how many volunteers will have to be reached in order to meet the randomization and retention goals. A funnel is an estimate of the number of volunteers who will drop out at each stage of the process—from the initial contact to the final close-out visit. Ideally, a statistician will estimate the drop-out rate up front—that is, the proportion of randomized patients who will complete the study. It is often left to the study managers to determine how many study volunteers will be needed to reach the randomization goal.

A funnel estimate should be completed for any phase II, phase III, or phase IV study. It enables study managers to estimate call center costs, the total number of site visits, and total screening costs. It will also help them determine if a centralized recruitment and retention company is needed to fulfill the study goals within the desired time frame.

Tracking Patient Progress

There are a number of places in which study volunteers can "fall out" of the study queue. Many will be disqualified because they did not meet the inclusion/exclusion criteria of the protocol. Others will find the study to be too time-consuming or intrusive and drop out. Still others will be poorly managed and drop out due to a lack of proper follow up or support on the part of the call center or study site. There are a number of reasons for patients to fall out. It is important to understand these and take action if a problem is identified. The following table shows the disqualification reasons provided by our call center for a recent study for the treatment of stress urinary incontinence.

Table 1: Pre-Referral Disqualifications

Disqualification Reason	Number	%
Disqualifying medication	2,611	12.6%
Surgery for urinary incont	2,474	12.0%
Incon not related cough sneez	2,141	10.3%
Not able to travel to site	1,885	9.1%
Treatment for heart disease	1,547	7.5%
Does not want to participate	1,191	5.8%
Treatment for neurological disease	1,111	5.4%
No site in area	1,026	5.0%
Body mass index	916	4.4%
Allergic reaction to sulfa meds	749	3.6%
No urinary incont symptoms	745	3.6%
No convenient site	714	3.4%
Surgery resulted in incont	692	3.3%
Gastrointestinal disorder	641	3.1%
BldPrsMeds changed w/in 3 mos	501	2.4%
Age	401	1.9%
Not willing to take birth control	338	1.6%
Uncontrolled high blood pressure	302	1.5%
Chronic obstructive airway disease	165	0.8%
Lactating	137	0.7%
Site threshold reached	112	0.5%
Alcohol abuse last year	96	0.5%
Other	66	0.3%
Uncontrolled diabetes	59	0.3%
History of thyroid disease	43	0.2%
Treated for bladder tumor	34	0.2%
End stage kidney disease	3	0.0%
Total disqualifications	**20,700**	**100.0%**

In a typical centralized recruitment scenario, advertisements are run on local radio, television, in newspapers and/or direct mail with a message that says "if you have a problem with _____ and would like to join a research study to test a new treatment, call 1-800-xxx-xxxx." The volunteers contact the call center, are given a pre-screen interview to determine if they are eligible for a clinical screening visit and (if they pass the pre-screen) are then directed to the study site closest to them. These are patient *referrals* If the call center is well-integrated with the sites and can schedule appointments on behalf of the sites while they have the volunteer on the phone, the volunteer does not have to make an additional call to the site to schedule an appointment (or the site does not have to contact the volunteer). This can have a great impact on the voluntary drop-out rate.

In the aforementioned stress urinary incontinence study, there were some sites that allowed the call center to set the initial appointment, and some that did not. It was found that when the call center was allowed to set the initial appointment, the site was able to...

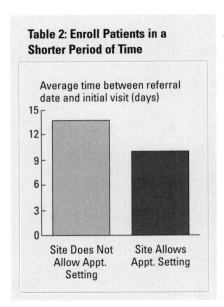

Table 2: Enroll Patients in a Shorter Period of Time

Average time between referral date and initial visit (days)

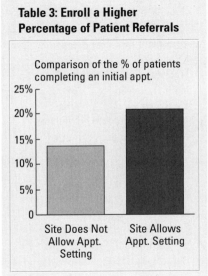

Table 3: Enroll a Higher Percentage of Patient Referrals

Comparison of the % of patients completing an initial appt.

These considerable differences in time-to-first-appointment and the appointment completion rate show that when the call center was not allowed to set the initial appointment, it had a significant negative impact on patient retention because it was left to the site or the study volunteer to follow up in a timely fashion to set the appointment. This created an added burden for both sides.

The example above demonstrates the importance of patient tracking. Qualified study volunteers can be very expensive to find. The advertising costs alone can run into the tens of millions for large-scale phase III trials. It can cost up to $1,000 in media costs to find a single volunteer who pre-qualifies for the study—that is, the *cost-per-referral*, can be as high as $1,000. One of the most common and costly mistakes that study sponsors make is to hire a stand-alone advertising agency to run their centralized campaigns.

Stand-alone agencies are not fully integrated with a call center or the individual sites. The agency will usually work from the call center reports and know how many callers and referrals are generated by their ads, but they rarely know what happens to those patients once they are referred to the nearest site.

In another study we ran television spots, radio ads, newspaper ads, and direct mail (the media mix depended on the market and a number of other factors). Within two weeks, it became clear that the cost-per-referral for newspaper was close to 40% higher than for the other media types. But as the study progressed, it was found that a much higher percentage of patients who were recruited via newspaper were randomized into the study. In fact, the cost per randomized patient was lower for patients recruited via newspaper ads than for the other media. Table 4 illustrates this point using dollar amounts that correlate to the actual figures, which cannot be divulged.

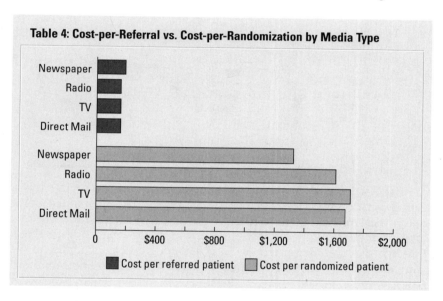

Table 4: Cost-per-Referral vs. Cost-per-Randomization by Media Type

Thus the patients who were recruited via newspaper were less expensive in the end than patients recruited from other sources. This illustrates the importance of system integration and effective patient tracking. If the media information is not fully integrated with the call center information and site data, the sponsor will never realize that it is paying more per randomized patient when it uses radio, TV and direct mail and will continue to run those ads. In fact, the sponsor may even drop the newspaper ads thinking they are too expensive.

Patients need a lot of attention to maintain their interest and participation. Many of them enter the trial to learn more about their disease or condition. They need to be educated about their disease, sent reminders of upcoming visits and have special needs accommodated (transportation,

upcoming visits and have special needs accommodated (transportation, rescheduling, etc.). This is particularly important early in the recruitment process when volunteers are feeling anxious and haven't fully committed to participating.

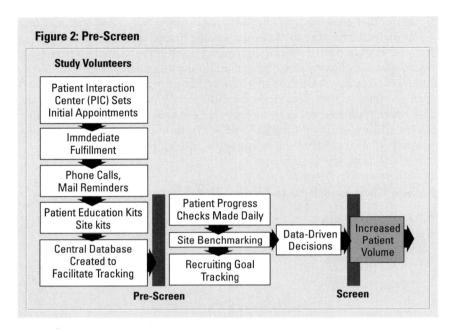

Figure 2: Pre-Screen

The best approach to retaining patients is to implement a multi-layered, data-driven review process that tracks their progress from their initial phone call to their final close-out visit. Once the patient is referred to a site, the sponsor needs to know if the site is actively following up with them. Research sites are often extremely busy, handling dozens of studies at the same time. If they are overwhelmed, the sponsor needs to know and take action by providing aid to the site, helping them follow up with patients, or reducing the number of volunteers sent to the site. This is one of the greatest challenges to centralized recruiting since the sites do not control the number of patients referred to them.

Monitoring Site Performance

The capabilities of study sites vary widely from small clinics with no Internet connection to large, technically savvy research institutions participating in 50 or more studies at the same time. Often, the study sponsor does not have a great deal of experience with some of the sites they have contracted for their trial. If it is not aware of what is going on with the volunteers sent to the sites, it can be months before the sponsor realizes that a particular site is not paying attention to their study—for whatever reason.

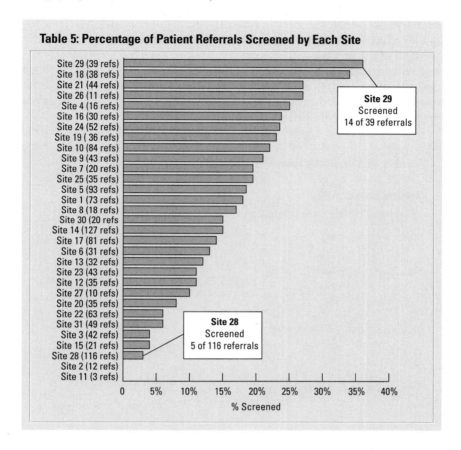

Table 5: Percentage of Patient Referrals Screened by Each Site

The histogram above is taken from a recent phase II trial to research a new treatment for type 2 diabetes. A centralized recruitment campaign was used to provide advertising and call center support to each of the local markets. The histogram shows the percentage of pre-qualified patients who were screened at each site. The number of pre-qualified patients sent to each site is shown in parentheses after the site identifier. The percentage of patients screened varies widely from 36% at Site 29 to 0% at Site 2 and Site 11.

Two sites are highlighted—Site 28 and Site 29. Site 28 was sent 116 pre-qualified referrals but only screened 5 of them. Site 29 was sent only 39 referrals but screened 14 patients—almost 3 times as many as Site 28. This example illustrates the challenges facing study sponsors who often struggle with the wide disparity in site performance.

Again, clinical sites are often very busy and can have months in which there is high staff turnover or an excessive workload (or both). These circumstances need to be understood and accommodated in the most judicious manner possible. If the problems persist for an extended period of time, it may be in the best interest of the sponsor to stop advertising in the site's market, and direct their media dollars to more efficient sites. The study team will not be able to ascertain where the problem areas lie, however, without an effective system of data collection and reporting.

If all of the sites have an Internet connection, it is usually efficient to collect patient status information using online forms. These form data are uploaded to a central database for compilation and analysis. The partial form below was used for the stress urinary incontinence study (complete forms include patient initials, address, etc.).

Figure 3: Patient Status Form (Partial Form)

Referral Date 6/9/2003

| Initial Appointment Date (mm/dd/yyyy) | Scheduled | 06/13/2003 |
| | Completed | 06/13/2003 |

| First Screen Visit (mm/dd/yyyy) | Scheduled | 07/07/2003 |
| | Completed | 07/07/2003 |

| Second Screen Visit (mm/dd/yyyy) | Scheduled | 07/29/2003 |
| | Completed | 07/29/2003 |

| Randomization Date (mm/dd/yyyy) | Scheduled | 08/11/2003 |
| | Completed | 08/11/2003 |

Disqualification Reason

Disqualification Comment

When merged with media information, site information and call center information, this comprehensive database becomes a powerful management tool to greatly enhance decision-making. The report howing the percentage of patients completing their initial appointment by age group (see Table 6) led us to redesign our communication strategy for older seniors who were "falling out" in greater numbers.

Table 6: Percentage of Patients Completing Initial Appointment by Age Group

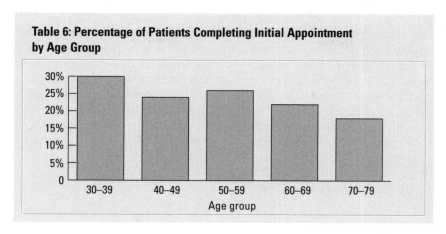

Setting Benchmarks and Projecting Results

The data collection tools described above enable the study team to drill down and make very informed decisions on a day-to-day basis. With the benefit of an online, real-time reporting system, they can set very specific goals and benchmarks and determine at any time how close (or far away) they are from them, site by site.

Phase II Study for Type 2 Diabetes

As mentioned, we recently managed a study for a new treatment for type 2 diabetes. The study participants had to be recently diagnosed and untreated, making this a very challenging group to identify and recruit. The sponsor had only been able to randomize 36 patients in the first eight months of the study, relying on the sites alone to find the patients and manage their

Table 7: Early Randomization Trend (Sites Alone)

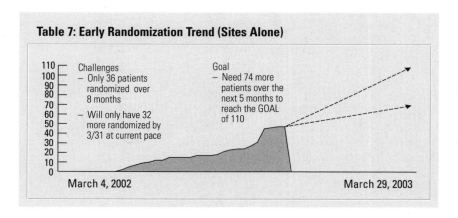

progress to randomization (not centralized) (see Table 7). This was well short of their goal of 110 by 3/31/03, which they simply had to reach, so they contracted us to accelerate recruitment and manage the study centrally.

Due to the upcoming holiday season, it was decided to run a small, two-week media test in a limited number of select markets to determine the effectiveness of the campaign (called WAVE 1). The media were successful, generating 426 pre-qualified patient referrals for the 16 sites (see Table 8).

One concern that arose from the test phase, however, was the length of time it was taking to get the patients scheduled for their visits. It was taking

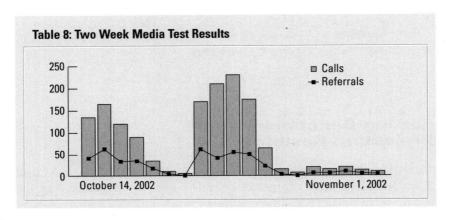

Table 8: Two Week Media Test Results

Table 9: Site Metrics vs. GOALS

Investigator	Number of Referrals	% of Referrals Completing their Initial Appt. within 14 days	ABOVE/ BELOW Target (18%)	Screen Comp
Site 1	73	25%	ABOVE	13
Site 2	12	25%	ABOVE	0
Site 3	42	2%	BELOW	2
Site 4	16	6%	BELOW	4
Site 5	93	5%	BELOW	17
...	...	...	...	...
Site 28	10	0%	BELOW	6
Site 29	116	17%	BELOW	6
Site 30	39	23%	ABOVE	14
Site 31	20	20%	ABOVE	3
Site 32	49	16%	BELOW	4
Total	**712**	**14%**	**BELOW**	**112**

the sites an average of 21 days to schedule and complete the initial appointments (two sites had delays in their local IRB approval). This was obviously too long, so a new training plan was implemented quickly to educate site staff more thoroughly on the data collection and patient management system. Benchmarks were developed to guide the site staff on the time requirements needed to reach the goal. Additional help was provided to sites with limited resources.

The second wave of media (WAVE 2) was launched right after the holidays in early January. The media campaign ran for five weeks in 28 markets

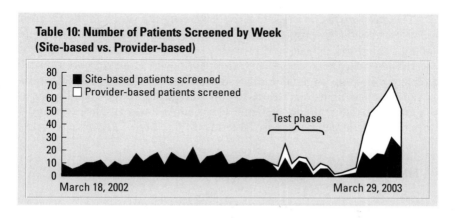

Table 10: Number of Patients Screened by Week (Site-based vs. Provider-based)

% Screened	ABOVE/ BELOW Target (15%)	Run-in Comp	% of Screened Pts in Run-in	ABOVE/ BELOW Target (50%)
18%	ABOVE	11	85%	ABOVE
0%	BELOW	–	–	–
5%	BELOW	1	0%	BELOW
25%	ABOVE	2	50%	ABOVE
18%	ABOVE	11	65%	ABOVE
...	...	...	...	...
10%	BELOW	1	100%	ABOVE
5%	BELOW	4	67%	ABOVE
36%	ABOVE	10	71%	ABOVE
15%	ABOVE	3	100%	ABOVE
8%	BELOW	4	100%	ABOVE
15.7%	**ABOVE**	**73**	**65.2%**	**ABOVE**

(supporting 32 sites). The trend in patient screening clearly jumped in January and February, and, more importantly, the sites were scheduling patients much more efficiently as can be seen in Table 10. Notice the elongated screening trend in the Test Phase versus the spiked screening trend in WAVE 2.

A number of reports were used to keep track of the pre-qualified referrals and the retention efforts at each site. These reports were made available to the sponsor and study team via the Internet and were accessible 24/7. One such report displayed the benchmarks for each site and ranked their progress, noting whether they were ABOVE or BELOW target.

These reports were very effective for keeping the sites and the sponsor well informed on the progress. They acted as an incentive for sites that were falling behind to catch up and provided positive recognition for sites that were doing well. These reports, in combination with active site communication and follow-up on patient status worked well in WAVE 2. The total time to randomize patients was reduced by an average of 12 days—mostly due to a significant reduction in the time to schedule and complete the initial appointments, as can be seen in Table 11.

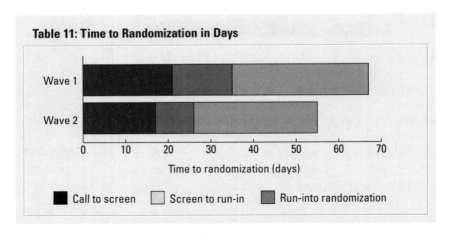

Table 11: Time to Randomization in Days

This management effort of benchmarking and monitoring progress was crucial to the success of the recruitment effort. After much nail-biting, we were able to exceed the randomization goal by 6 patients before the deadline.

In the very competitive and often frenetic world of clinical trials, the level of management described in this chapter has to be applied to optimize success. As was pointed out in the beginning of the chapter, the financial stakes are high and the patients are expensive to find. It is simply not feasible to expect success in the face of these mounting challenges—particularly in the U.S. marketplace—without a well-designed study program including recruitment strategy and tactics that have demonstrated success.

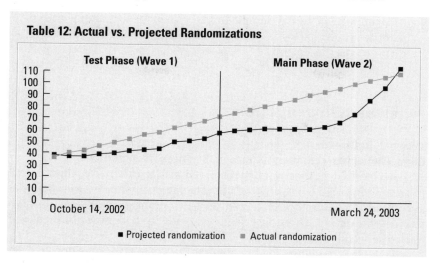

Table 12: Actual vs. Projected Randomizations

(Test Phase (Wave 1) and Main Phase (Wave 2); y-axis 0 to 110; x-axis from October 14, 2002 to March 24, 2003. Legend: ■ Projected randomization, ▪ Actual randomization)

Summary

Patient recruitment and retention for clinical trials has become very fragmented and expensive. Delays in patient recruitment can cost study sponsors millions in lost revenues. For larger trials, site-based recruiting has proven to be very unpredictable and difficult to manage. When executed properly, centralized recruiting offers significant economies of scale and more control over the projected recruitment outcomes. Study benchmarks and metrics drive the success of a well-executed centralized recruitment and retention effort.

Key Takeaways

Data-driven programs helped us determine that:
- A higher percentage of patients are enrolled—and enrolled faster—when the call center is allowed to set appointments
- The cost-per-call is not an adequate measure for determining media spend for each market. The cost-per-randomization or cost-per-completion should ultimately drive media decisions.
- Sites vary greatly in their capabilities and performance levels. Sponsors need to be able to recognize poor performance quickly and rapidly adjust strategy.
- Site benchmarks can be used to significantly affect performance—such as reducing the time from referral to initial appointment completion.

■ Media testing in a small sample of markets enables the study team to identify problem areas at low cost and maximize the effect of subsequent media placements.

Author Biographies

Kathleen B. Drennan
Chief, Global Marketing and Strategic Business Development
As a recognized authority on pharmaceutical research and clinical trial processes, Kathleen Drennan develops integrated support services that offer significant opportunity in pre- and post-marketing clinical trials through brand optimization. Those areas include worldwide patient recruitment and related services.

Ms. Drennan, known for her ability to leverage business opportunities through recognizing best-fit alliances, partnerships and acquisitions, developed the first academic, for-profit, centralized clinical research organizations for Rush-Presbyterian-St. Luke's in Chicago and for the University of Pittsburgh Medical Center. Under her leadership as founding President and Chief Operating Officer of The Chicago Center for Clinical Research, CCCR became one of the largest and most successful independent trial organizations in the country. CCCR developed performance-based strategies that led to the successful implementation of more than 100 significant clinical trials annually and has been used as the model for clinical research. Previous to her CCCR tenure, she spent eleven years at Upjohn Pharmaceutical Company in cardiovascular research and development.

Investigators and industry, alike, have attended her workshops and presentations for over eighteen years spanning a variety of topics, including cost-management of clinical trials, business strategy, clinical operations development and women's health. She is published and highlighted for her accomplishments in a variety of trade magazines and scientific journals, including the *Wall Street Journal, Crain's Business, Modern Physician, Applied Clinical Trials, Women in Medicine* and *PharmaVoice*. Her most recent article, published in *Pharmaceutical Executive*, features her analysis of current industry challenges.

Ms. Drennan has recently been appointed Editor-in-Chief for Elsevier's international journal, *Controlled Clinical Trials*.

As founding member of the Society for Women's Health Research in Washington, D.C., she currently presides on their Board of Directors. In 1995, Ms. Drennan was inducted into the University of Illinois' Entrepreneurship Hall of Fame, sponsored by William Blair & Company, Arthur Anderson Enterprise Group and LaSalle National Bank.

Jonathan Bailey
Director, Analytics and Statistics

Jon Bailey is currently the Director of Analytics & Statistics for Iris Global Clinical Trial Services, and principal architect for Iris' database, reporting, metrics and modeling systems. His expertise was sharpened over 15 years of "hard knocks" with pharmaceutical and health industry leaders such as Pfizer, Aetna and the Coordinating Center for Biometric Research—and technology leaders like Dell and InfoWorks. He has authored numerous white papers and articles on statistical system design, optimizing patient recruitment and retention, and maximizing ROI. Jon holds an M.S. in Biostatistics from the University of Minnesota.

A B O U T   T H O M S O N   C E N T E R W A T C H

Thomson CenterWatch is a Boston-based publishing and information services company that focuses on the clinical trials industry and is a business of the
Thomson Corporation. We provide a variety of information services used by
pharmaceutical and biotechnology companies, CROs, SMOs and investigative
sites involved in the management and conduct of clinical trials. CenterWatch
also provides educational materials for clinical research professionals, health
professionals and for health consumers. We provide market research and market intelligence services that many major companies have retained to help
develop new business strategies, to guide the implementation of new clinical
research-related initiatives and to assist in due diligence activities. Some of our
top publications and services are described below. For a comprehensive listing
with detailed information about our publications and services, please visit our
web site at www.centerwatch.com. You can also contact us at (800) 765-9647
for subscription and order information.

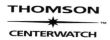

22 Thomson Place · Boston, MA 02210
Phone (617) 856-5900 · Fax (617) 856-5901
www.centerwatch.com

CenterWatch Training and Education Manuals

The Investigator's Guide to Clinical Research, 3rd edition
This 250-page step-by-step manual is filled with tips, instructions and insights for health professionals interested in conducting clinical trials. *The Investigator's Guide* is designed to help the novice clinical investigator get involved in conducting clinical trials. The guide is also a valuable resource for experienced investigative sites looking for ways to improve and increase their involvement and success in clinical research. Developed in accordance with ACCME, readers can apply for CME credits. An exam is provided online.

How to Find & Secure Clinical Grants
This 28-page guidebook is an ideal resource for healthcare professionals interested in conducting clinical trials. The guidebook provides tips and insights for new and experienced investigative sites to compete more effectively for clinical study grants.

A Guide to Patient Recruitment and Retention
This 250+ page manual is designed to help clinical research professionals improve the effectiveness of their patient recruitment and retention efforts. Written by Diana Anderson, Ph.D., with contributions from 18 industry experts and thought leaders, this guide offers real world, practical recruitment and retention strategies, tactics and metrics. It is considered an invaluable resource for educating professionals who manage and conduct clinical research about ways to plan and execute effective patient recruitment and retention efforts.

The CRA's Guide to Monitoring Clinical Research
This 400-page CE-accredited book is an ideal resource for novice and experienced CRAs, as well as professionals interested in pursuing a career as study monitors. *The CRA's Guide* covers important topics along with updated regulations, guidelines and worksheets, including resources such as: 21 CFR Parts 50, 54, 56 & 312 Guidelines, various checklists (monitoring visit, site evaluation, informed consent) and a study documentation file verification log. This manual will be routinely referenced throughout the CRA's career. Developed in acccordance with ANCC, readers can apply for CE Credits. An exam is provided online.

eClinical Trials: Planning and Implementation
This invaluable resource is designed to assist biopharmaceutical companies, CROs and investigative sites in understanding, planning and implementing electronic clinical trial (eCT) technology solutions to accelerate and improve their research operations. Written by highly respected thought leaders in the field today, this 180+ page book describes and addresses the concepts and

complexities of managing and conducting an optimal eCT, while offering practical guidance, facts and advice on implementing eCT technologies.

Protecting Study Volunteers in Research, Second Edition

This second edition of our top-selling manual has doubled in size to address current and emerging issues that are critical to our system of human subject protection oversight. *Protecting Study Volunteers in Research* is a suggested educational resource by NIH and FDA (source: NIH Notice OD-00-039, 2000, page 37841, Federal Registry 2003, page 47342) and is designed to help organizations provide the highest standards of safe and ethical treatment of study volunteers.

Developed in accordance with the essentials and standards of the ACCME. Readers can apply for up to 6.5 CME credits. Developed in accordance with the essentials and standards of the ANCCC. Readers can apply for up to 7.8 Nursing Contact Hours. An exam is provided with each manual.

Evaluating the Informed Consent Process

This 12-page booklet reviews the results of a recent survey conducted among more than 1,500 study volunteers. This booklet presents firsthand experiences from study volunteers and offers valuable insights, facts and data on the informed consent process and how this process works.

Online Directories and Sourcebooks

The Drugs in Clinical Trials Database

This database is a comprehensive web-based, searchable resource offering detailed profiles of new investigational treatments in phase I through III clinical trials. Updated daily, this online and searchable directory provides information on more than 2,000 drugs for more than 800 indications worldwide in a well-organized and easy-to-reference format. Search results may be downloaded to Excel for further sorting and analysis. Detailed profile information is provided for each drug along with a separate section on pediatric treatments. *The Drugs in Clinical Trials Database* is an ideal online resource for industry professionals to use for monitoring the performance of drugs in clinical trials; tracking competitors' development activity; identifying development partners; and identifying clinical study grant opportunities.

The eDirectory of the Clinical Trials Industry

Previously available as a printed directory, the new *eDirectory* is a comprehensive, online, searchable and downloadable database featuring detailed contact and profile information on 1,400+ organizations involved in the clinical trials industry. Company profiles can be searched by keyword, company name, city, state, phase focus, therapeutic specialties and services offered. Search results can be downloaded to an Excel spreadsheet for further sorting and analysis.

Profiles of Service Providers on the CenterWatch Clinical Trials Listing Service™

The CenterWatch web site (**www.centerwatch.com**) attracts tens of thousands of sponsor and CRO company representatives every month who are looking for experienced service providers and investigative sites to manage and conduct their clinical trials. No registration is required. Sponsors and CROs use this online directory free of charge. The CenterWatch web site offers all contract service providers—both CROs and investigative sites—the opportunity to present more information than any other Internet-based service available. This service is an ideal way to secure new contracts and clinical study grants.

An Industry in Evolution, 4th edition

This 250-page sourcebook provides extensive qualitative and quantitative information documenting clinical trial industry trends and benchmarked practices. The material—charts, statistics and analytical reports—is presented in an easy-to-reference format. This important and valuable resource is used for developing business strategies and plans, for preparing presentations and for conducting business and market intelligence.

CenterWatch Compilation Reports Series

These topic-specific reports provide comprehensive, in-depth features, original research and analyses and fact-based company/institution business and financial profiles. Reports are available on Site Management Organizations, Academic Medical Centers, Contract Research Organizations, and Investigative Sites. Spanning nearly seven years of in-depth coverage and analyses, these reports provide valuable insights into company strategies, market dynamics and successful business practices. Ideal for business planning and for market intelligence/market research activities.

CenterWatch Shopper!

The *Shopper!* focuses on specific products and services and presents them in a compelling format designed to make it easier for you to compare them and to select the best options for your business needs. Experts and thought leaders contribute tips and pointers to assist you in considering and evaluating various product and service offerings.

CenterWatch Patient Education Resources

As part of ongoing reforms in human subject protection oversight, institutional and independent IRBs and research centers are actively identifying educational programs and assessment mechanisms to use with their study volunteers. These initiatives are of particular interest among those IRBs that are applying for voluntary accreditation with the Association for the Accreditation of Human Research Protection Programs (AAHRPP) and the National Committee for Quality Assurance (NCQA). CenterWatch offers a variety of educational communications for use by IRB and clinical research professionals.

Informed Consent™: A Guide to the Risks and Benefits of Volunteering for Clinical Trials

This comprehensive 300-page reference resource is designed to assist patients and health consumers in understanding the clinical trial process and their rights and recourse as study volunteers. Based on extensive review and input from bioethicists, regulatory and industry experts, the guide provides facts, insights and case examples designed to assist individuals in making informed decisions about participating in clinical trials. The guide is an ideal educational reference that research and IRB professionals can use to review with their study volunteers, to address volunteer questions and concerns, and to further build relationships with the patient community. Professionals also refer to this guide for assistance in responding to the media.

Volunteering For a Clinical Trial: Your Guide to Participating in Research Studies

This easy-to-read, six-page patient education brochure is designed for research centers to provide consistent, professional and unbiased educational information for their potential clinical study subjects. The brochure is IRB-approved and is used by sponsors, CROs and investigative sites to help set patient expectations about participating in clinical trials. *Volunteering for a Clinical Trial* can be distributed in a variety of ways including direct mailings to patients, displays in waiting rooms, or as handouts to guide discussions. The brochure can be customized with company logos and custom information.

A Word from Study Volunteers: Opinions and Experiences of Clinical Trial Participants

This straightforward and easy-to-read ten-page pamphlet reviews the results of a survey conducted among more than 1,200 clinical research volunteers. This brochure presents first-hand experiences from clinical trial volunteers. It offers valuable insights for individuals interested in participating in a clinical trial. The brochure can be customized with company logos and custom information.

Understanding the Informed Consent Process

Understanding the Informed Consent Process is an easy-to-read, eight-page brochure designed specifically for study volunteers. The brochure provides valuable information and facts about the informed consent process, and reviews the volunteer's "Bill of Rights."

The CenterWatch Clinical Trials Listing Service™

Now in its ninth year of operation, *The CenterWatch Clinical Trials Listing Service™* provides the largest and most comprehensive listing of industry- and government-sponsored clinical trials on the Internet. In 2003, the CenterWatch web site—along with numerous coordinated online and print affiliations—reached more than 10 million Americans. *The CenterWatch Clinical Trials Listing Service™* provides an international listing of more than 42,000 ongoing and IRB-approved phase I–IV clinical trials.

CenterWatch Newsletters

The CenterWatch Monthly

Our award-winning monthly newsletter provides pharmaceutical and biotechnology companies, CROs, SMOs, academic institutions, research centers and the investment community with in-depth business news and insights, feature articles on trends and clinical research practices, original market intelligence and analysis, as well as grant lead information for investigative sites.

CWWeekly

This weekly newsletter, available as a fax or in electronic format, reports on the top stories and breaking news in the clinical trials industry. Each week the newsletter includes business headlines, financial information, market intelligence, drug pipeline and clinical trial results.

JobWatch

This web-based resource at www.centerwatch.com, complemented by a print publication, provides comprehensive listings of career and educational opportunities in the clinical trials industry, including a searchable resume database service. Companies use *JobWatch* regularly to identify qualified clinical research professionals and career and educational services.

CenterWatch Content and Information Services

Market Intelligence Reports and Services

With nearly a decade of experience gathering original data and writing about all aspects of the clinical research enterprise, the CenterWatch Market Intelligence Department is uniquely positioned to provide a wide range of market research services designed to assist organizations in making more informed strategic business decisions that impact their clinical research activities. Our clients include major biopharmaceutical companies, CROs and contract service providers, site networks, investment analysts and management consulting firms. CenterWatch brings unprecedented industry knowledge, extensive industry-wide relationships and expertise gathering, analyzing and presenting primary and secondary quantitative and qualitative data. Along with our custom research projects for clients, CenterWatch also facilitates on-site management forums designed to explore critical business trends and their implications. These sessions offer a wealth of data and a unique opportunity for senior professionals to think about business problems in new ways.

TrialWatch Site-Identification Service

Several hundred sponsor and CRO companies use the *TrialWatch* service to identify prospective investigative sites to conduct their upcoming clinical trials. Every month, companies post bulletins of their phase I–IV development programs that are actively seeking clinical investigators. These bulletins are included in CenterWatch—our flagship monthly publication that reaches as many as 25,000 experienced investigators every month. Use of the *TrialWatch* service is FREE.

Content License Services

CenterWatch offers both database content and static text under license. All CenterWatch content can be seamlessly integrated into your company Internet, Intranet or Extranet web site(s) with or without frames. Our database offerings include: *The Clinical Trials Listing Service*™, *Clinical Trial Results*, *The Drugs in Clinical Trials Database*, *Newly Approved Drugs*, *The eDirectory of the Clinical Trials Industry*, and *CW-Mobile* for Wireless OS® Devices. Our static text offerings include: an editorial feature on background information on clinical trials and a glossary of clinical trial terminology.

Continuing Medical Education (CME) Symposia

Continuing medical education (CME) symposia feature a variety of useful and practical topics for clinical research investigators, study coordinators, CRAs, clinical research scientists, physicians and allied health professionals. Thomson CenterWatch has developed flexible, turn-key programs that can be integrated into investigator educational settings in order to promote higher levels of compliance and study conduct performance.

NOTES